SURVIVAL END GAME

The 21st-Century Solution

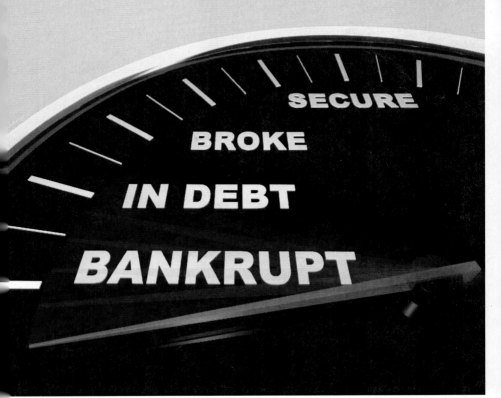

Paladin Press • Boulder, Colorado

Also by Ragnar Benson
Acquiring New ID
Do-It-Yourself Medicine
Eating Cheap
Guerrilla Gunsmithing
Live Off the Land in the City and Country
Mantrapping
Modern Survival Retreat
Modern Weapons Caching
Most Dangerous Game
Ragnar's Action Encyclopedias, Volumes 1 and 2
Ragnar's Guide to Interviews, Investigations, and Interrogations
Ragnar's Guide to the Underground Economy
Ragnar's Tall Tales
Ragnar's Urban Survival
Survivalist's Medicine Chest
Survival Nurse
Survival Poaching
Survival Retreat: A Total Plan for Retreat Defense
Switchblade: The Ace of Blades: Revised and Updated (with Michael Janich)
Ten Best Traps . . . And a Few Others That Are Damn Good, Too

Survival End Game:
The 21st-Century Solution
by Ragnar Benson

Copyright © 2013 by Ragnar Benson

ISBN 13: 978-1-61004-861-3
Printed in the United States of America

Published by Paladin Press, a division of
Paladin Enterprises, Inc.
Gunbarrel Tech Center
7077 Winchester Circle
Boulder, Colorado 80301 USA, +1.303.443.7250

Direct inquiries and/or orders to the above address.

PALADIN, PALADIN PRESS, and the "horse head" design
are trademarks belonging to Paladin Enterprises and
registered in United States Patent and Trademark Office.

All rights reserved. Except for use in a review, no
portion of this book may be reproduced, stored in or
introduced into a retrieval system, or transmitted in any
form without the express written permission of the publisher.
The scanning, uploading, and distribution of this book by the
Internet or any other means without the permission of the
publisher is illegal and punishable by law. Please respect the
author's rights and do not participate in any form of electronic
piracy of copyrighted material.

Neither the author nor the publisher assumes
any responsibility for the use or misuse of
information contained in this book.

Visit our website at www.paladin-press.com

CONTENTS

Introduction		1
Chapter One	**What Hasn't Changed**	5
Chapter Two	**Knowing What Is Ahead**	11
Chapter Three	**Survival Relocation**	19
Chapter Four	**Water**	29
Chapter Five	**Finding Value During the Collapse**	39
Chapter Six	**Three Sources of Food**	49
Chapter Seven	**Energy**	59
Chapter Eight	**Shelter**	67
Chapter Nine	**Security**	75
Chapter Ten	**Medical**	83
Chapter Eleven	**Equipment and Supplies**	91
Chapter Twelve	**Employment and Retirement Relative to the Rule of Threes**	101
Conclusion		109

To Pete and Pat Warwick, without whose quiet, competent, reliable assistance this volume would have been mostly impossible.

PREFACE

Fortunately there is really nothing new under the sun. From stoic, traditional Japan, which has been in economic recession for 30 long years, we can note that its survival still pretty much mirrors what we thought was our old, familiar pattern here in the United States. However, and this is a big however, we learn from modern Greece, Spain, and Italy that violent, unthinking, counterproductive mob reaction to forced austerity is the new standard response. How does it help individuals or society in general for violent mobs to burn down stores simply because owners have no funds to maintain an inventory of goods for sale to the public at prices the mob determines to be "fair"?

Valid economic fixes are out there, but increasingly citizens won't tolerate them.

Longtime readers of my works on survival realize that I have made a life's work of observing and understanding survival in many different nations and societies around the world, up close and dirty. These have included everything from primitive mud-hut survival in such places as northern Kenya, Somalia, and Burma, to urban survival in Hiroshima, Beirut, Cairo, and Havana.

Having now, as of this writing, spent anywhere from 3 1/2 weeks to 3 1/2 years in 95 different places around the world, I feel confident that my experiences and observations can be instructive and valid for "overcomer-type survivors."

It is also important to note that I have lived as a survivor for more than 50 years during my time at my U.S. home. Theory, this book is not. I eat my own cooking and have personally seen it all through the years in numerous places around the world. All the remedies herein have been tried and tested. My report follows.

INTRODUCTION

Any time someone claims that "this time it is different," be very suspicious. This assertion is often made about everything from child rearing to investing to managing some kind of enterprise to surviving, but it is seldom true. Events and technology do change but, in my experience, not terribly frequently.

Economically, it wasn't different in the mid-1990s during the dot.com panic. Recall this as a time when investors claimed—with a straight face and really no larceny in their hearts—that insisting on a salable product that made profits in the market was an obsolete concept for companies. Without profits, thousands of business enterprises collapsed when no new angel investors stepped forward. All of a sudden, it really was all about producing something of value at a profit.

It was not much different for food producers when new, overly strict rules and regulations precluded the use of laborsaving, cost-efficient production technologies. Predictable results were easily seen in our supermarkets as food prices—especially for fresh produce—spiked dramatically. As always, increased costs tied to decreased unit production led to price increases. Even the agricultural industry discovered that this time it really wasn't different.

There was no difference for American workers who insisted on even higher wages, benefits, and pension plans. Now priced out of the market, they watched in dismay as their jobs disappeared into lower-cost markets overseas. Nothing new or different there either.

College and university students who thought that this time was different ran up high education bills in preparation for low-paying jobs. Now, with no prospect of paying their tuition bills, they do know (or should know) that this time it *wasn't* different, after all. But try to explain that to Occupy Wall Street folks.

And the list goes on and on. There is nothing different about the necessity of buying a house you can actually afford to make payments on or, on an international basis, expecting a tax-spend-regulate economy to bring on prosperity. Although many Americans are seeing through these subterfuges, folks in Greece, Spain, and Italy still cannot make themselves realize that this is the road to ruin, not prosperity. Plenty of prior examples exist, but these folks can't see them. For these and many other reasons, we must proceed very cautiously into any new survival strategy.

It is pretty tough to admit I was wrong, especially given good examples of London and the entire United Kingdom, Paris, Tokyo, and Berlin after World War II. Madrid, including all of Spain after its civil war; Argentina; Cuba; Mexico; and Burma after its most recent economic collapse, are all good examples of practical survival strategies that are no longer entirely valid. With the exception of Cuba, most of these are examples of societies that quickly and efficiently went about surviving their most-recent traumas, eventually leading to a new and bright future. Not without blood, sweat, and tears, including great loss of life to be sure, but the survivors in these places provided good, workable lessons for us to study and apply to our own survival. They illustrate examples of large groups of people who simply accommodated the inevitable, including their current situations. They quietly did what they could, accepting what they had to, and eventually prevailed.

Humans are, by nature, quick to learn, often very stoic, and accommodating—or at least have been until the current era. Think of the collapsed, grave economy in Iran in this regard. Using these examples, building a workable survival plan was relatively straightforward. Not easy, but straightforward. It is important to note that these earlier dislocations were viewed as temporary. And if not temporary, emigration was always an option . . . a luxury current survivors no longer enjoy.

Introduction

Day-to-day details of how exactly to survive haven't changed that much, but external realities weighing on the survivor and his family have changed tremendously. I include much more about this in following chapters. Yet we do have a great many good examples of modern survival to work with. For example little Iceland has some extremely valuable lessons for us to note, especially the importance of having rural roots to fall back on in an economic crisis.

One of my bankers is not especially given to philosophy. His day-to-day experiences with people under economic stress have led him to some interesting, even shocking, conclusions. Four really big problems facing our society, as he sees them, compromise our future and our children's future, our economy, and our entire society. Summarizing dramatically, these include the fact that average Americans today seem to firmly believe that:

1. "I deserve it."
2. "It's not my fault."
3. "I want it now."
4. "It is someone else's responsibility to provide goods and services—probably the government's."

This is exactly the mindset currently tearing apart Greece, Spain, and Italy.

As a result, 21st-century survivors who really want to be overcomers must reorient their entire thinking to include a great deal more obscurity, defense and personal responsibility, and production—all while simultaneously preparing for what currently seems to be a very long and arduous haul.

Past survival mentalities, which focused on preparations for a relatively short term or just until the crisis had passed, are no longer workable, especially for those who insist on staying in cities.

Having finally admitted to ourselves that, against all odds and historic logic, things really have changed this time, we must proceed in a somewhat different fashion. Americans still have a few economic options now completely closed to the Greeks,

French, Portuguese, Spaniards, and Italians. But sooner is still better to take action. So, we must get on with our preparations while we still have those options available to us.

CHAPTER ONE

WHAT HASN'T CHANGED

Other than some very large issues—such as the fact that survivors must now plan for the very long term, probably including great changes in lifestyle and occupation, as well as the fact that functioning survivors will be heavily pounced on by government-supported citizens who wish to "appropriate" their goods—what in your necessary survival skills repertoire *won't* change?

Many small changes in your survival means and methods will evolve, but a good number of major skills and procedures we learned or planned on learning as 20th-century survivors are still valid. Perhaps you should substitute "necessary" for "valid."

When in Russia a few years ago, I asked a rural peasant farmer about the survival "rule of threes." The good fellow lightened immediately, quickly confirming that this was certainly part of the rural Russian mentality—one that they continue to follow while living out their lives. But I was surprised when the fellow emphatically corrected me on its origin. It wasn't invented by Russian farmers, as I had thought, but rather it came from the Russian Orthodox Church, having to do with its teaching on the Holy Trinity. Quickly disclaiming any knowledge of the exact origin of this concept, I told him that it was now a bedrock concept of American survival and preparedness planning.

Reviewing a bit, the rule of three tells us that there aren't very many essential components for life in a survival situation. But for the vital few, we must realize that, without them, life ceases—quickly and cruelly. As a result, thorough preparation must be made for three distinct sources of supply for each of these vital elements. In many cases, these three sources should include at least one that is renewable. All sources should be reliable, not theoretical. Walking over to a lake a mile away for your water supply is a good example of a theoretical supply source that may not be valid or workable. Hardscrabble survivors actually in the game will quickly find that supposed secure sources are anything but. You might initially plan to use a resource if after diligent research it seems reliable, but later in actual practice you have to be prepared if it proves not so. It's why we plan for three in each case. Exactly like the Russian who decided it was essential that his pants not come down, so he wore a belt and suspenders and sewed buttons on his shirttails to tie to his pants, making sure those pants stayed in place. That is the rule of threes in practice.

Absolute essentials for life constitute a very short list. They include food, water, energy (which may be a subset of others), shelter, and medications. Without these in adequate and timely amounts, life will be short, brutal, and painful. Some real-life survivors also list a category called "self-actualization" or "comfort items." This includes such items as reference sources, school supplies or toys for the kids, Bibles, books for pleasure reading, music, or maybe some favorite pieces of art. Reviewing the experiences of Russians in their gulags suggests these items really can be significant to long-term survival. Details providing for and defining these items are found in the following chapters. Also note that there are many subsets of these items, as well as some unavoidable overlaps.

Providing these few essential items requires a dramatic increase in personal responsibility and self-reliance for most citizens. Decreases in government rules, regulations, and oversight lead to potentially greater prosperity in the long run but are extremely hard on those who cannot accept greater freedom and its attached elements of greater personal responsibility on the part of the individual.

Bottom line? If you, the survivor, do not provide for these items, you must assume that nobody else will. We should also note that provision of these necessities must be made in a timely manner. In other words, start now while impending crises are still looming, not after they are under way.

To summarize, a drink of water the morning after you die of thirst isn't really any sort of promised-for water—it really isn't even a drink of water. During the 1930s, European Jews had a window of opportunity to survive, but by the early 1940s survival was no longer an option for most of them. Likewise, most Greeks, other than those few still on small rural farms, may have waited too long to act for survival to be likely. It may also be true for the Spaniards and Italians. France has no hope. In the case of Ireland, they are still pretty much rural, and Iceland is still overwhelmingly rural. People in the United States and Canada still have a bit of time to come up with a survival plan and start to implement it.

History has shown that survival is a grueling business, often entailing more than 14 hours per day at dull, repetitive tasks. That has not changed, nor will it in the future. Effective survivors must mix modern technology with ancient techniques. Think of the importance of providing lights to augment short winter days in our northern hemisphere. A generator and light bulbs may be vital to your long-term survival. Oil-lamp purists might not fare as well. Whenever possible, you should plan to use modern fuel-efficient devices, such as high-efficiency light bulbs and LED flashlights. Yet another modern example may be including the use of a freezer or freezers to preserve and store vital food supplies.

Another universal, unchanging lesson best looked at now relates to levels of comfort individual survivors may demand or tolerate. Perhaps you should prepare by dialing the heat down to the high 50s in your retreat and augmenting with a couple of warm sweaters and wool pants, or incorporating enough freeze-dried food for several years into your current food budget. But you say you cannot tolerate itchy, scratchy wool clothing, and that you don't like cheap, bland, easily stored but nutritious dried beans, peas, rice, and lentils? You'd better settle these types of issues now while you have time to make accommodations.

Purchasing enough freeze-dried food for several long years, or even a decade, is not an option for most survivors because of the expense. So how do you work around this? It is just as important to store the right types of food as to put away adequate amounts. It might be safer for you to choose dull, routine foods that you look forward to only when you are very hungry. That way you are not tempted to dig into your limited food supply out of laziness.

Conservation of energy is another important universal rule of survival. Proper survivors never violate this rule, which simply states that you must never expend more energy in pursuit of supplies than is earned by that activity. Under certain circumstances, examples may include sport hunting, cutting firewood by hand, gathering wild edibles, hauling water, manufacturing vital repair parts by hand, using a hand-crank generator, or even using a bicycle. I'm not saying that these activities are necessarily counterproductive, but they may be too inefficient to ensure long-term survival on their own. You have to figure this out based on your situation.

Too many folks in our society think it would be cool to go back to pre-machine-age methods of producing things. They fail to factor in the time and energy required to do such tasks, at a time when every ounce of energy and every second of time will matter. It is vital to quickly identify time and energy sinks before they bankrupt survivors. There is no place for Luddism in your survival plan. Your goal is doing whatever it takes, using whatever resources you have available to prevail in the most timely, efficient manner possible.

As a result, survivors must carefully inventory their future requirements, setting aside vital tools, spare parts, supplies, and equipment against the day of need. I discuss this much more in the following chapters. It is sufficient at this point to know these constraints still apply.

An extremely skilled computer technician came to see me about joining a survival group. He had accurately read the tea leaves and was anxious to make a plan for his family and himself. I asked him what usable skills he possessed—was he a good, if not expert, welder, machinist, trapper, gardener, butcher, generator technician, or something else? His response was, "I fix computers." My response was that I can't see that as a reliable skill of interest or use to survivors. He stormed out in anger.

Contrast his reaction with that of a top-of-the-line, extremely clever Jewish attorney who also saw pervasive signs of our society's demise and wanted to become part of a survival group. Right from the start the fellow admitted he had no survival skills.

"How long would it take you to become expert at chain saw repair and maintenance?" I asked.

After a bit of thought, he responded, "Perhaps four to six months, and I believe I could do a credible job."

No wonder he was a good attorney. His ability to think through tough situations was exemplary, as was his willingness to adapt.

Even the American Indians each had separate, distinct skills, according to my Uncle Dugan, a full Ojibwa. Some members of his tribe were hunters, some trappers, some gatherers, some food processors, and so on. Together they survived because of their mix of skills.

Survivors cannot escape the basic truth that they absolutely must have at least one skill—and preferably three skills, again the rule of threes comes into play—related to their circumstances. In proper settings, skills may be traded, but you've got to have something of value to trade. This is an ironclad rule, which may seem overly obvious to some of you, but maybe not to many others who are just starting out.

Summarizing, workable survival plans that have not changed in the 21st century:

- Always use the rule of threes.
- Always take into account conservation of energy.
- Avoid the lure of economic or social purity. You must incorporate modern techniques into your survival plans as appropriate and necessary.
- Be aware that you will have to downsize and adapt a great deal, likely including some level of suffering.

- Know that with irreplaceable supplies, such as food, boredom can play a significant role. Survivors may be best served by storing mundane, cheap, nutritious foods that they will consume slowly and not gobble up.
- Tremendous amounts of preplanning and personal responsibility will be required. Note that I use the word *required* not *helpful*.
- Survivors must have usable skills with which to maintain their retreat and to trade with others for needed products or services.

CHAPTER TWO

KNOWING WHAT IS AHEAD

Looking at countries around the world whose problems are similar to our own but far more advanced, we can accurately see what lies ahead. Unfortunately, seeing "what" is a far cry from knowing "when." Fortunately, we also now have a means of predicting when. This involves a method that has always been with us but has only recently come into sharp focus: the close monitoring of government bond rates, as discussed on page 16.

Other good news for alert survivors is that, although we may not know exactly when, our predictions for the future will give us some additional time to prepare. Like bankruptcies, financial crises leading to collapsed societies happen slowly, slowly, slowly . . . until the very end when the collapse occurs in a big hurry. Survivors need to know how to recognize when we are close to the "big hurry" stage.

Our first example is Japan, whose economy has been sick to very sickly for the past 30-plus years. Citizens there prove that collectively humans try very hard to adapt, no matter how tough their circumstances. In a nutshell, that's why predicting exactly when is tough to do (but not impossible, as we shall see). Adapting has a definite downside. Rather than correcting problems by decreasing government rules and regulations—along with shrinking bureaucracies, taxes, and spending while increasing personal responsibility—Japanese people just quietly go along. Culturally, it may be impossible for them to change, no matter how severe their problems.

The European community provides additional examples. Shortly after taking over as prime minister of the United Kingdom in 1979, Margaret Thatcher strongly resisted taking the UK into the European Common Market. She accurately predicted that the European Union (EU) could not survive: "Of the bureaucracy, for the bureaucracy, and to the bureaucracy. This beast cannot live on."

We don't know Prime Minister Thatcher's predicted time span for how long the EU could survive, but now—some 25 years later—we see that it is indeed experiencing great problems living on. Similar to individual humans, the Europeans tried very hard to adapt to a very bad deal. "Kicking the can down the road" is a term many Europeans (and Americans) use to describe putting off the inevitable in the hopes that the problem will either go away or be handled by someone else.

Rather than doing away with economically strangling edicts on a massive scale, European leaders hold one unproductive, self-seeking conference after another. Italians have raised this activity to an art form. Currently Italian labor laws make it impossible to start and grow a company in Italy. There is no such thing as vital foreign investment in that country, much less any internally generated growth.

Greek citizens react by burning buildings, shutting down vital tourist industries, rioting in the streets over unpaid pensions, and vilifying Germans who won't continue to make Greek welfare payments. At the same time, Greek citizens who are unable to flee their troubled land are relegated to bartering for fuel and medications already in such short supply that they are almost nonexistent. (Another lesson here is that there is nothing wrong with barter on a personal scale if survivors are prepared for it.)

A massive amount of what little money remains is flowing out of Greek banks and into German, Swiss, and Scandinavian banks, further impoverishing Greece and adding to the need for a barter economy. Both Greece and Spain are experiencing tremendous deflation. Prices for food, clothing, hotel rooms, and many personal services are falling like a wounded vulture.

Evidence from Greece also alerts us to the fact that survivors still around for the last phases of a collapse will face some extremely strange government actions calculated to collect more money. Bureaucrats in Athens, for instance, slapped a tax on electric bills. I am not making this up. Rather than privatizing electric companies, thus cutting expenses, salaries, and pensions, the Greek government tried to raise people's vital expenses at a time when residents had absolutely no means of paying. Currently in Spain, federal law dictates that government employees cannot be fired even when there is no money to pay salaries. Go figure . . .

France, under its new regime, is trying higher taxes and increased spending, along with significantly more rules and regulations. By time of publication, readers can judge for themselves how well this is working out for the French.

Thus, we can see that at the same time that salaries and business profits are crashing, government officials are attempting to raise taxes. Perhaps the European folks really do have a reason to riot.

Two English couples and a German couple, each coming to the United States to visit for the first time, remarked that our media has done a horrible job of explaining how things really are here. They expressed the opinion that CNN does an especially awful-to-dishonest job. "Nothing they report is accurate," they told me. I suggested that they look at another channel, but their point is one also currently echoed by Greeks, Spaniards, and Italians: no accurate news is available from their TV programs or newspapers.

Survivalists had best prepare for this to happen to them. In some cases, we will be able to accurately know a few things, but generally there will be a news blackout wherein bad news is denied or glossed over or bad news is artfully spun into "good news." We can hope that independent sources on the Internet will distribute accurate information in the United States, but we shouldn't count on it. And will the Internet even be available to survivors? Perhaps not.

We must also be aware, based on EU experience, that our money may buy little, if we can even access it. This is different from having our money debased by inflation, which was the scenario traditionally expected by survivors. Vendors in a few places in Europe—including Greece, Cyprus, Iceland, and to some extent Ireland—are not accepting currency of any kind.

The important lesson here is that significant portions of the American population still believe we can tax, spend, and regulate our way to prosperity. We in the United States are, at this writing, looking at the effects of a financial crisis that has led to higher taxes with no real cuts in spending. No matter how this plays out, it won't have a good effect on our economy. But there is no sense in getting into that debate here.

Cutting taxes and increasing spending to stimulate the economy no longer work, as evidenced by our recent experience in the United States. Only massive amounts of in-depth deregulation of the type we saw under President Reagan in the 1980s, Gerhard Schröder in Germany in the late 1990s and early 2000s, and Margaret Thatcher in the United Kingdom in the 1980s will work. But there is not much sign of that happening in many places around the world, much less in the United States. A few indications of deregulation of a very preliminary nature exist in a few places. About 3,000 small business rules and regulations were recently abolished in England. Additionally, Spain, Greece, and Italy are actually relaxing ruinously high minimum wage rules to some limited extent.

However, in Spain, Italy, and Greece today, individual effort leading to personal accomplishment is said to no longer work. Those remaining are demoralized. We can only hope that this attitude will not infect many American survivors. The fact that people can no longer expect to retire on time (or at all) certainly applies to Americans. In that regard, we should expect our ranks of survivors to be swelled by great numbers of bewildered Americans who believed that their overly generous yet underfunded pensions would eventually materialize. Angry protests in Wisconsin on the part of public service employees who saw their unsustainable pensions diminished is a good close-to-home example of this.

Will these folks eventually hunker down, making good, viable survivors? Only time will tell. Yet we do know that, in their urge to get reelected, politicians the world over have dramatically overpromised their citizens. That's something all of us can continue to count on. Overly enthusiastic promises of the good life without accompanying economic production happened not only in Greece, Spain, Italy, Portugal, France, Ireland, Iceland, and Cyprus, but also throughout most of the developed world. Iceland and Portugal provide special lessons in that regard.

Portuguese citizens are not rioting over their country's obvious bankrupt state. Perhaps because they so recently emerged from a brutal dictatorship, Portuguese citizens simply resign themselves to sucking it up again. Also, Portugal tends to be still a bit more of a rural-based society. Moving back to the farm with Mom and Dad doesn't seem that drastic to many of them.

Iceland provides another excellent example, at least for now, of a small, unique, basically rural land that seems to have pulled itself back from the abyss. Here lessons for American survivors abound. First, Iceland is almost entirely a rural country with only one large city. It is also a small, tight-knit, culturally homogenous society with a strong history of cooperation and self-reliance. Going back to living with one's parents on a small, isolated station where they ate fish they caught, ducks and geese they shot or trapped, greenhouse vegetables they grew, or sheep and cattle they raised is not considered a hardship. Most Icelanders still live very close to the land. Icelanders pride themselves on the fact that they did not cut welfare payments or collectively reduce wages. That they halved the exchange value of the krona, effectively paying everyone half as much as before and doubling prices of imports, seems to have flown right by most citizens.

The above examples of those who fared best in Portugal and Iceland strongly suggest that survival anyplace but out in the country in our 21st-century context will be extremely difficult.

Now comes the important part, referenced at the start of this chapter: how survivors can predict with some degree of accuracy the collapse of their society. There is a way. The mechanism has always been there but only recently come into full view. It's not the advent of rioting and demonstrations that always seem to break out when it becomes painfully clear that governments cannot provide the good life they promised. These riots and demonstrations can signal the "slowly, slowly" part that precedes a sudden collapse. Prudent survivors must learn to watch government bond rates, *both* state and national, as well as total national and state debt. Catastrophic rates are not set in concrete, yet when *they* approach or exceed 6 percent, this strongly suggests there is great trouble on the horizon, along with a need for great caution and more earnest preparations on the part of effective survivors.

Current economic crises in Europe, Cuba, Argentina, and Venezuela—as well as in California and Illinois—followed high bond rates. What these high rates tell us is that it now takes more borrowed money to pay for government largesse and to service debt than is being taken in by taxes. Governments now have to pay more money to fund interest on both new and existing debt than they are collecting. A lot of this depends on high levels of unretired historic debt *and* debt levels that begin to exceed all national economic activity. In other words, when total government debt exceeds total national production, 6 percent interest rates quickly kill an economy and its society. Many countries currently must borrow money to pay interest on current borrowing.

Estimates vary dramatically, but we in the United States probably aren't quite there yet. However, including state and municipal debt, we are perilously close to 100 percent of GNP. Doubters will claim that borrowing in this country currently costs about half of our 6 percent interest trigger point. This is true, but principally because our government is printing and circulating massive amounts of money. We don't see inflation because we are not spending that money. There are too many people out of work or seriously underemployed, along with a great many folks scared into great caution. Massive personal-debt reduction is now under way, as citizens pay down credit card debts or walk away from delinquent home loans. Unfortunately, our leaders have not gotten the message regarding national debt.

Why don't Americans see this looming crisis? Some do, but they are too few and too powerless to do anything about it. And significant numbers can't think their way out of this situation. There are also a bunch of folks sucking on the tit who are going to ride the economy into the ground and get as much as they can while the getting is good. Another group of thinkers genuinely believe that when more than one-half of voting citizens are on the government dole, collapse is inevitable. Examples abound.

Obviously Occupy Wall Street folks flunked fifth-grade math, yet they may be representative of many Americans. So we should not expect enough citizens to notice, believe, or act on bad bond data. Yet coupled with the fact that national and state debt exceeds gross national product, the data is out there for those who want to survive.

I know that this is a gloomy, horrible assessment, but it is one based on realities seen in our current world. And I see nothing on the horizon that will make things better, chiefly because most powerful politicians are either stupid, short-sighted, or bound by other agendas. But we can know the tipping point, making proper preparations to survive and perhaps prosper feasible. That is the lesson of this chapter.

CHAPTER THREE

SURVIVAL RELOCATION

This is the chapter I really did not want to write. It is probably the most difficult because many good, otherwise like-minded folks will either not want to believe or will choose not to act on this information. Some may even become hostile.

Think back to European Jews during the early 1930s. As mentioned, they had a pretty good idea what was coming, but most elected to stay in Europe, where they intended to survive the coming storm. As a result, millions lost everything, including their lives.

Recommendations here are based on a great deal of study of both current situations and historic ones. Since this is the bitter pill, I have elected to eat the live toad now, putting this difficult chapter toward the front of the book so that nothing worse will follow. Significantly, the problems we now face have changed from those encountered in past crises. In fact, they have changed dramatically. In times past, we could be reasonably confident that horrible conditions faced in large and medium cities would improve, often fairly quickly. This time around, we must conclude that we are definitely in this for the very long haul—probably four to six years, and some smart people even suggest 10 years!

As a result, we cannot continue to rely on measures calculated to see us through an especially tough six to eight months, after which our food, water, energy, and shelter situations will start to improve. Even out in the country, it will be very difficult to store enough of everything for a four- to six-year run. Even if you could afford cash outlays for such, spoilage and deterioration over so great an interval would wipe out most of us. We must think of resupply in much expanded terms, *which is only reasonable out in the country.*

For example, take the issue of vital electrical power in cities. If your power goes out—as is common in Greece, Cuba, and Italy—what to do? Fire up the emergency generator for your fourth-floor apartment? Probably not. How are you going to keep the neighbors from being involved? Where will the necessary fuel come from? How do you hook it up? What about noise, smells, and perceived pollution? Survivors in Beirut, Lebanon, during that nation's civil war made great use of little Honda gas generators. But folks using them were camped on ground floors, and they were always short of fuel. A clandestine market eventually developed, providing some fuel. Yet, it was not one survivors could really count on.

As a result of the "I am deserving," "I want it now," and "you must have stolen from poor people to enjoy the goods you now have" attitudes, defending your retreat will be a very big issue. This is a huge game changer that does not seem solvable in cities.

Currently people in Greece, Italy, Spain, and Ireland complain bitterly about the lawlessness that has recently welled up in their societies. Theft and plunder, previously uncommon, have become rampant. Municipalities outside the capitals have no money for police. Most of those few officers remaining do so only because they demand and take huge bribes. There is no local money for anything, much less fuel for police cars. Wise observers note that local municipalities frequently go broke well before state and federal authorities. In the United States, that is also true today in parts of Michigan, Illinois, and California, to name only a few states.

Trying to personally maintain law and order in large cities is frequently not possible or practical in today's world. Those who have come to expect and demand the good life provided by others have demonstrated that they will not hesitate to take what they want from others, by force if necessary. Especially if takers perceive that those they plunder have achieved the relative good life they are living by subterfuge and dishonesty. Shooting someone in defense of yourself or your property will most likely bring down the wrath of what's left of society, led by citizens jealous of your preparations and preparedness.

Lawlessness aside for a moment, cities in collapsed economies quickly become very unhealthy. Consider how rapidly diseases will spread with no garbage collection, few medicines or trained medical professionals to treat people, and no maintenance of sanitary disposal and water supply. Diseases, rats, and insects will multiply. Municipal water, drains, and sewers will fail with no one to fix them. Such is now becoming more and more evident in Athens.

Then there is the overwhelmingly serious matter of reliable, potable water. During World War II, residents of Moscow, Berlin, and Dresden hauled their water home from fetid rivers and puddles, often from great distances, after municipal supplies were cut off. In Soviet Russia water workers were sent to death camps when they could not repair water mains without replacement pipes. In many European cities, benevolent occupiers brought in water trucks to rescue urban dwellers. No benevolent suppliers are on the horizon this coming go-round.

What often isn't remembered about World War II is the extent to which many city people still alive after a few months quickly departed. Distant acquaintances out in the country frequently found on their doorsteps long-lost second cousins or friends they knew only vaguely. And those people who did remain in cities profited immensely from being only a generation or two removed from the farm. They already knew how to keep rabbits on the balcony, raise vegetables in the parkways, and harvest leaves from linden trees. Such is definitely not true today among city dwellers.

Whether you want to hear it or not, those who leave now for a new life in the country have the option of taking most of their goods with them, rather than fleeing by foot under great duress in the middle of the night with perhaps a bug-out bag and little more. Other than in infrequent situations on the part of some very few, very fortunate, and very rich city people, only country folks will survive. Your choice is to go rural now in good order or go later under great duress.

Some of you may be thinking that with the large number of people trying to relocate to rural America and the limited amount of land available to them, the rural areas will quickly fill up. Certainly, this concern is a valid one. However, my experiences in Spain, Greece, Cuba, and Japan convinced me that most people will actively choose to remain in the cities. It seems that small towns gain population but do not fill up. For a great many years now, people have left small rural towns and farms for big cities. Quite a large number of people can return to the countryside before any real problem occurs. People in both Iceland and Portugal returned to their rural roots in relatively large number during their financial upheaval. It is important to note that they had rural roots to return to, something painfully lacking in the United States these days.

Frequently refugees don't even know where they are headed—just anyplace away from the starvation, mayhem, anarchy, and disease around them in the cities. A survival rule of thumb suggests that once you become a refugee, you are as good as dead. You may survive for a while, but a slow, painful death is likely.

More bad news for urban dwellers is that while property values in cities have suffered, for the most part rural properties have maintained their value. Farmland is selling at record highs, largely because of record-high crop prices. Folks in newly prosperous small towns have bid up the prices of modest homes on an acre or two. Throw in a small barn and prices start to look like really big bucks. Therefore, few real estate bargains exist in rural areas.

An important survival principle is that people do poorly with debts hanging over them. This is true even when the economic conditions are favorable, but debt becomes even more burdensome during an economic meltdown. While not universally true, financial institutions in some places have become oddly and unpredictably more aggressive about collecting amounts owed them, and at times even before these debts are due. Folks struggling to afford food and water do not need this additional pressure. For the most part in imploding societies where salaries and employment in general are unpredictable, a good rule of thumb is to have no significant family or personal debt after age 50. I know that's a tough rule to follow, but as mentioned at the beginning, this is a tough chapter. No debt after age 50 was an item of faith for the Amish folks among whom I was raised. Does anyone doubt that these folks will survive nicely *without* any additional preparation?

When evaluating potential rural retreat sites, keep firmly in mind that every rural area in the United States (and perhaps most of the world) faces the threat of at least two potentially devastating national disasters that city people may not expect or understand how to deal with. A very short list of these potential disasters would include regional fires, floods, avalanches, wind storms, tidal waves, extreme cold or deep snow, ice storms, earthquakes, droughts, and disease epidemics. Wise newcomers to rural areas should make diligent, in-depth inquiries about the occurrence of these phenomena in the past. Of course, people can and do live through these catastrophes, but they do so much better with prior knowledge and preparation.

Securing proper title to rural land and amenities is another commonly overlooked pitfall. Long personal experience strongly suggests that as many as half of the rural parcels available may not be situated as described in the title, or the titles themselves may be so poorly executed that they are next to worthless. Often this just reflects lax standards rather than outright dishonesty. I can think offhand of a carport built out in the middle of a platted right of way and a fence erected 30 feet to the east of a property line, robbing the neighboring property of significant acreage and a spring. After finding property that suits your needs, go to the expense of having it properly resurveyed, thereby locating all the corners. Ask neighbors about easements and other anomalies that could arise. Also talk to county officials, title companies, assessors, county road and highway personnel, and bankers. Actively pursue every lead. Don't rely solely on a local attorney to do your own research.

Be especially cautious regarding zoning restrictions. Some

longtime residents resent newcomers they don't know, leading to a "the answer is no—what's the question?" mentality. A humble, open attitude will help identify and then overcome potential problems.

Also be certain about underlying mineral rights. Our current oil shale boom has exacerbated this problem, making prior sale of mineral rights a much more widespread and serious issue than it once was. One survivor, whom I know well, wisely backed out of a somewhat large property deal on discovering that oil drillers could access his property any time, any place, without any warning whatsoever!

You must also be certain about water rights, especially in the West, and easements that may halt or restrict use of that specific property. These restrictions could be critical during a survival situation, affecting your access to water, what you may build on the property, and whether the land can be fenced off and secured. Detailed talks with as many locals as possible are again important here, with two objectives in mind: convince locals you are a nice, valuable, nonthreatening addition to their community; and find out about potential glitches and problems before you commit to a property. This research is time consuming and difficult, but it must be done.

Survivors should move only to rural places that are productive agricultural areas and where they know they can tolerate the climate. Let's take agricultural issues first. While most city people cannot accurately evaluate soil types, fertility, and land-carrying capacities, there are simple, straightforward indicators for neophytes. Look at areas or entire regions with many *active,* large steel or cement grain storage silos or tanks, both on farms and at grain terminals in regional centers. These indicate that large amounts of corn, wheat, soybeans, oats, barley, and other grains are being produced, stored, and perhaps shipped out from the immediate area. (It is vital that you ascertain that the silos are currently being used for grain storage; in some areas big grain elevators or silos have been unused for years or repurposed for other uses, which won't help with your food resupply. Usually

Survival Relocation

these have been replaced by on-farm storage, or grains are shipped right from the field to export facilities. The important thing to note is that grains are being grown locally.) Also note the presence of potato or onion storage cellars, as well as hog and cattle feedlots or chicken barns.

Farmers likely will not be able to engage in large-scale agricultural production if our crises deepen, adding materially to the disruption. This would occur as a result of a lack of fuel, seed, chemicals, feed supplements, and fertilizers. Sustainable agriculture without a reliable source of fuel, seeds, and chemicals cannot feed all of us. But this is a book about personal survival, and even though the bins may not be filled every year, some food will be produced that survivors might barter for or purchase. Farmers are generally very proactive and resourceful. As an example, Cuban farmers went back to using horses and oxen during their collapse period, and essentially this is what is happening in rural Greece and Portugal today.

American farmers might not resort to such measures on a large scale, but the determined among them will continue to cultivate their land and produce some food products. And alert, smart, prepared survivors can supplement their food requirements from this production. Using field corn, wheat, or barley raised for livestock for human consumption will present a significant challenge, as I have found few really tasty methods of preparing these commodities. Survivors who learn to exist on these crops will definitely not gain weight!

Fuel is another big issue with modern farmers. I personally am aware of at least four farmers who have on-farm storage facilities for 30,000 gallons of number 2 diesel fuel. Will they part with some small part of this to aid local survivors? Only time will tell what sort of relationships can be built before the time of need arrives. A lot depends on how soon you start developing relationships with your neighbors.

Climate is another great consideration before choosing a new area in which to relocate. Right now there is time to get it right. Be certain your vision is not one of heading off into the deep, dark woods up north to live in a chop-out hole. Several people recently have told me that is their plan. It is not a realistic one if their intent is staying alive or avoiding a long, slow, cruel death.

Visit areas you have in mind during all four seasons. Every season is slightly different every year, but visitors can get some sort of idea of what to expect. Is there a sufficient growing season? I know of two areas only two miles apart where growing seasons vary by a full 100 days! Are winters livable as well as workable? Weather charts from local realtors can help, but it is better to talk with potential neighbors about what they grow in their gardens and what that entails.

Often this subject provides a bitter, difficult choice. Close friends are retreating near Bakersfield, California. Weather and climate for them are very positive: put seeds in the ground, and they grow year-round. Yet politically the area is not compatible for survival-oriented people, and it has severe issues with water. These two factors are probable game changers for most survivors. Access to water will be covered in depth in the next chapter, but be aware that in many areas availability of water is a tremendous issue. Both you and your garden require regular drinks of the stuff when nature turns off the spigot. Our friends in Bakersfield are absolutely convinced that California is no longer a democracy and that financially and socially the state cannot survive. Valid relocators must keep these types of factors in mind, regardless of how perfect the physical climate is.

Back to gardening. Most likely all survivors will have to learn how to garden. Maybe you have a black thumb, and gardening as a source of replaceable food for you is not practical. The only way to know for sure is to find out now before being overtaken by a coming crisis. Do your research and make an earnest effort to grow a garden. Work at it diligently. If you fail, some potential exists in a few places for you to glean produce after truck or farm harvests. However, you should not count on this source, as commercial harvests will be interrupted in many areas. And, of course, some nongardening folks can trade goods or vital skills for local farm food.

Gardening is not the only source of food for survivors, of course. Collecting wild edibles is one possible source, but at least initially for most new survivors this is insufficient as a food source. All areas have their natural wild bounty there for the taking, but gathering and using swamp cattails, acorns, and other foraged foods require knowledge of the plant life in the area you will be inhabiting. For example, what parts of the plants can be safely eaten (and when), and how do you prepare them? This is another area where you will be required to do your research well before a crisis arises. And you have to keep in mind the conservation-of-energy principle: are you exerting more energy stalking wild edibles than you are gleaning from consuming them?

Shooting or trapping ducks, geese, deer, turkeys, raccoons, squirrels, or rabbits might appeal to you as an option for procuring food, but it may currently be outside your skill set. Even if an area provides bountiful opportunities, they may not be reliable or accessible to you. It's the same with keeping cows, pigs, chickens, or goats. This is wonderful in theory, but can *you* do it successfully? Again, these skills must be learned over time.

Another factor to consider when relocating is privacy. You should look for a place where it is possible to be anonymous and hidden from view. Keeping a low profile is the only true defense against being plundered that survivors can count on during these perilous times. Fortunately, robbery is not as prolific in rural areas as it is in cities, though it could get worse if people are desperate.

How about sources of fuel for cooking and heating the retreat? Are these available in the areas you are considering? Are they renewable or, at the very least, replaceable?

A category often overlooked by those evaluating a rural retreat location is a source for any special needs you might have. These can range from auto and tractor mechanics, septic tank services, and medical treatment and supplies, including stitching up really horrible accidental wounds. All these examples are from personal experience. Many city people just assume these services are not available in rural areas. In *all* cases, city newcomers will be shocked by numbers of highly skilled, self-trained, sometimes unlicensed rural people available to help with your special requirements.

In one recent, very notable instance, a fellow brought his 9-, 10-, and 11-year-old sons to help on a difficult emergency roofing job on a steep, three-story rural barn. This would not be possible in big cities with numerous inspector-type scolds, yet they banged out a tough job in less than a day.

Of course, caution is required here. Our area supports one of the finest backwoods, seat-of-the-pants, informal parts makers ever to set foot on this Earth. The fellow is brilliant and very skilled. However, he is extremely picky about for whom he does any work. If you are a socialist or a racist, don't count on this fellow's help.

Merchants and business people claim there are only three really important elements of success: location, location, location, in that order. The same is true with survivors. The importance of finding an area that will support you and your family cannot be overemphasized. The vital necessity of familiarizing yourself with the economic and political environment, seasons, and events in your new home and of starting now is the primary takeaway of this chapter.

CHAPTER FOUR

WATER

I made every attempt in this book to list vital survival/preparedness requirements in order of priority. The short list of essential items includes water, food, shelter, energy, and medications. Absent any of these, life ends quickly. No priority exists, readers quickly note. Dead is dead.

True enough, yet without adequate clean water you will go to your reward much, much faster in an incredibly more miserable fashion. Think of the prospects of passing from terminal diarrhea caused by rough, wiggly water!

Significantly, securing clean, adequate supplies of water quickly points us to one of the new game-changing elements of 21st-century survival of which we must be aware: the grim fact that governments do not want their citizens to be independent or self-reliant. Survivors are looked on with fear and suspicion, subject to instant regulation. Not being dependent on government aid and services for all your day-to-day requirements is an incomprehensible concept to many citizens and most bureaucrats. This seems true no matter who is in power or where you are in the world. Regulators everywhere seem pathologically insistent on putting more and more rules and regulations in place, severely limiting your ability to be responsible for your own well-being. Personal responsibility has become a foreign concept that is looked down on with fear and loathing.

With water, this dramatically expanding regime of onerous, foolishly restrictive rules and regulations is becoming especially severe. It seems that, unless you move quickly, it may become impossible to "legally" secure sufficient water on which to live.

You think this an exaggeration? At this writing, the federal Environmental Protection Agency is trying mightily to remove the word "navigable" from the U.S. Clean Water Act. By so doing, it would allow federal bureaucrats to regulate and control even roadside ditches and culverts that only occasionally hold water briefly after a rainstorm. Think this wouldn't affect you? Once the federal regulators have secured the ability to regulate and to issue permits, I see no end to federal intrusion, including the use of water from small streams, domestic wells, and anything that diverts water—perhaps even swamp water—for domestic use. Any private use of a small spring could, for instance, be impossible without costly and difficult-to-obtain permits.

Changing administrations seems of little practical value. Once these new super-intrusive rules and regulations are enacted, they take on a life of their own. Very few are ever repealed or forgotten. Most, if not all, remain in the background until citizens either forget about them or learn to live with them. Then selective, arbitrary enforcement becomes a wicked tool of the bureaucratic enforcers. Examples abound.

Currently some states already make it illegal to divert natural rainfall off your own house or barn roof into storage tanks or a cistern unless the property owner also has the groundwater rights. It is tough to see how this regulation could be effectively enforced, unless used arbitrarily and capriciously to control survivors. This is part of the brave new world survivors now face in many Western states, such as Oregon, where these rules are being enforced vigorously. (Colorado passed laws in 2009 that made private collection of rainwater legal in most instances.)

Collecting and saving rainwater for future use in fiberglass tanks, barrels, or even regular special-built cisterns might be one part of a water rule of threes you put in place. Other sources of water may be more practical or efficient, yet saving water for future use is often one part of a survival water plan.

As a brief aside, some nice, modern, sturdy, light, and easily handled fiberglass tanks with 300- to 500-gallon capacity are currently available at modest prices from agriculture-supply stores.

Should survivors conclude that storage is one of their water rules of three, such tanks would fit nicely into that program.

Making the best use of runoff rainwater also requires that you engineer your gutters and downspouts in such a way that the water can be collected efficiently. Laying back sufficient suitable plastic tarps and barrels should also be part of your water-collection strategy.

Many rural properties already rely on wells or some other developed means of providing potable water. Access to water is almost always why the locations of rural houses and farmsteads were selected in the first place.

Some states, principally in the West, are beginning to license or require permits for small private wells. Required filing for limited water rights could also be a future problem. Small-scale, domestic, rural water wells might continue to fly under regulatory radar for a short time yet. In many cases, delivery of municipal water in rural areas has made these wells redundant, which means that survivors could reactivate and clean their existing but currently unused wells as a backup in case of emergency. Owners might have lost their water rights to these wells, but who will know—other than the survivor—that these wells are back on line?

Clean an old, unused well by dumping a gallon of common bleach down the pipe, wait two days, and then pump for several hours or till the water level is drawn down. In all cases, survivors relying on personal wells must have an extra pump and spare parts in their supplies. This might entail buying two new pumps, as existing ones in old wells will probably have seized up.

It may also be possible in your rural area to have a new, full-scale, functional well drilled. Regulations regarding size and output may restrict your choice, yet it may be possible by choosing a smaller domestic well. This is another area of inquiry and research you will need to pursue.

Drilling large, deepwater wells can be expensive. Some cost-saving devices are out there, yet conventional wisdom teaches us that well drillers—like attorneys—happily work along until all our money is gone!

Extensive, early, diligent inquiry must be made relative to water when considering an area for a survival retreat. Relative to water and to the rule of threes in general, this is the most important concept.

Areas where water levels rise up to within 30 feet of ground level are inexpensively and quietly adaptable to driven or small-augered wells. Driven wells involve a procedure wherein property owners purchase special well points and heavy-duty 1.5-inch iron pipe that can be pounded down into the ground to water level. Suction pumps only work to about 30 feet, limiting their use if water levels do not rise to this level in well pipes. Effective submersible pumps are not made for small 1.5-inch wells.

Local plumbing shops and neighbors can usually supply good information regarding whether this old-fashioned, primitive method is workable in your area. Driving a well by hand is a very old-fashioned technique that many folks may have forgotten.

Another very inexpensive method of bringing in an inexpensive water well involves using a small, hand-operated, gasoline-engine-powered auger machine. You auger down about 30 feet and then quickly slip a 1.5-inch pipe into the hole.

Even where extensive expensive permits are required, either pounding down a driven well, finding the right person to auger a well, or even purchasing a well auger machine can quietly lead to a significant new source of survival water.

Specific instructions on how to drive or auger a modest new well are beyond the scope of this chapter. It is sufficient to say it can be done and that there is a lot of online information available to survivors. Technically, there is quite a trick to it. I am sure many of these little wells are still being installed daily in the United States, especially in the Midwest and South.

Frequently rural properties are located near a spring rather than a bored well because they were ruinously expensive during the early 1900s when many rural properties were settled. Flowing springs are simple courses of underground water moving along on top of an underground layer of impermeable clay or rock. They often originate miles and miles from their outlets.

Springs are developed for domestic use in rural areas by digging a modest holding area with a small dam at the end of the holding basin so filling and a bit of storage occur. Sometimes this holding place is simply a hole in the ground. More sanitary and permanent development can be made by building a cement tank or inserting a plastic or fiberglass basin in the collection hole. A length of plastic pipe is inserted into the dam wall, reaching into the tank below the permanent water level. Usually, but not always, this plastic pipe runs downhill from the spring to a larger, more sanitary collection tank near the homestead. Systems of this sort operate effectively on small islands in Alaska's Aleutian chain, especially where spring output per hour is miniscule but adequate over longer periods.

Spring water is usually cold, clean, and crystal clear, though contamination can be introduced at the catch basin. As a result, many springs are developed using containers in the catch basin, as well as by building roofs over the initial collection areas.

Water taken from a nearby lake, river, or stream may or may not require filtering and decontamination. Many rural folk simply pump water from deep within a lake or river, using it as it comes. But you would have the know the area and what may or may not be polluting the water to determine whether this is safe.

Local and national authorities may not like the fact that you are using "their" lake, spring, or river water. Yet, in many rural areas, survivors may easily get by for four to six years before anyone notices or takes action. Almost every rural house in the lake districts of northern Wisconsin and Minnesota is supplied by lake water.

Many purchased water systems come with built-in filtration and purification systems. Improvised water filters can easily be made as needed for spring, river, lake, or swamp water. Construct a shallow, hollow frame of 2 x 4s. Fill this with sand or fine gravel. Running water through this sand- or gravel-filled frame onto a plastic tarp that funnels into holding containers takes out large lumps. Cloth towel, hot tub filters, and such like may also be used as filters.

While this procedure removes large lumps, it will not filter microscopic organisms that can lead to disabling diarrhea or other waterborne illnesses. The easiest method of killing microorganisms in clear (not muddy) water is by using bleach. Since most survivors will not have to rely on rough water that must be treated for long periods, most will be able to sustain life for four to six years by laying in an inexpensive supply of calcium hypochlorite, a powerful pool cleaner sold commercially as "Pool Shock." The advantage of storing calcium hypochlorite instead of bottled bleach (e.g., Clorox or Purex) is threefold: it is much cheaper, it requires much less storage space, and it has a much longer shelf life, as opposed to liquid bleach which has an effective shelf life of three to six months before its effectiveness is diminished.

A 16-ounce bag of calcium hypochlorite costs about $4.00, and the chemical is often available at full-service plumbing supply stores, as well as pool-supply centers. The 16-ounce bag will make about 1,000 pints of chlorine bleach, which in turn will disinfect up to 10,000 gallons of water. The correct ratio to make a chlorine solution is one teaspoon (about 1/4 ounce) of calcium hypochlorite granules to two gallons (eight liters) of water. *Do not drink this solution; it must be diluted.* To disinfect the water, add one part of the solution to 100 parts of water. After sitting for about 30 minutes or more, the water is now safe to drink. If the water has a pronounced chlorine taste, aerate it.

My family's three-part water program consists of a deep well, stored runoff water, and stale, yucky pond water. We hope we never have to use the pond water, but we are prepared if the need arises. It also might be possible to safely slip into town to fill a 250-gallon fiberglass tank from time to time. (Most rural communities have public places where potable water can be purchased and hauled away. While this facility may not be available in an emergency situation, inquiring now certainly won't hurt.) The emphasis here is on "might." This last source is sufficiently questionable that it is not included in our rule-of-three water plan.

Humans require about two gallons of water per day per person for personal consumption and use. Throw in a quick shower every other day, laundry, food preparation for storage, cooking, and flushing toilets, and we are up to about five gallons per day, per person, at a minimum.

Obviously survivors will not water their lawns, but gardens must be maintained. In many areas of the United States, this means that watering may be required during at least part of the growing cycle. In arid or semiarid areas or during prolonged droughts, gardens may have to be watered several times a week. How much water is needed for the garden is unknown until you work out exact amounts for your specific needs. A local survivor, for instance, pulls water from a local intermittent stream into a tank truck for use on his garden. He is sure that exactly 6,000 gallons per season is his requirement. Another gardener planted over an underground stream in an area characterized by only seven inches of rainfall a year, so he never has to irrigate.

Recently a popular instructive travel magazine ran an article claiming that half of American travelers to Third World countries developed some form of travelers' diarrhea! Some knowledgeable observers postulate that average Americans are especially subject to stomach upsets because we currently tend to live in superantiseptic societies and are infrequently exposed to common bacteria. Necessary resistances are then never established.

Having now lived and worked in a great many Third World countries, I have only once—40 years ago—picked up traveler's diarrhea, in Mexico when I first traveled there. This is in spite of the fact that I have never been overly vigilant.

Abundant irrigation water taken from open canals and ditches is sometimes thought of as a potable water supply. Because this water is so extremely seasonal, it may present an occasional opportunity but never one to rely on year-round. An extended stay in your retreat will fully demonstrate the fickle nature of ditch water. However, water drawn from closed irrigation wells may provide a reliable supply. Some irrigation water is pumped from rivers, lakes, and reservoirs. This water may also be usable. Only diligent inquiry will tell.

Sanitary disposal is only partly about water, but where else do we consider this survival necessity? Burnable trash can be collected to be burned during cold times to heat your retreat. Resulting ash should be used as a source of vital micronutrients to spread on gardens, meadows, or forests.

Burying degradable garbage in the garden is often faster and more convenient than composting. Resulting improvements to soil structure and fertility are often dramatic.

Cans, bottles, and other trash items usually diminish in types, number, and amounts not long after serious retreating begins. Huge piles of trash can easily compromise a retreat, so take caution with finding a good method of disposal. Survivors may easily find themselves victims of especially desperate and stringent rules and regulations. It is probably best to continue to use landfills until later in a crisis. Then some plan for quietly and unobtrusively burying these items may be implemented. There is no possible way to deploy these methods for city retreaters.

Septic disposal is another very big issue for retreaters. Your fallback may be a simple two-hole outhouse, but this remains a giant "may be." Even in some rural locations, stringent rules and regulations prevent the use of old-fashioned outhouses.

Home-built, expedient, short- and medium-term septic systems are relatively quick and easy but, of course, violate tons of rules and regulations. As kids and young adults first moving into our own new houses, we buried two 55-gallon barrels for use as septic tanks. The first barrel caught and digested solids, while the second barrel, connected at the top with two-inch pipe, was the liquid holding tank. A 300-foot length of buried drain field pipe carried off all wastewater as the second tank filled. Some of these simple, cheap systems provided good service for 10 years or more. In especially arid areas, placing wastewater on or under the garden is wise but, of course, not always practical.

Simply burying 300 to 500 feet—space permitting—of drain field pipe also works as a septic system. Sewage decomposes in the pipe and eventually is leached into the drain bed. These sorts of systems are highly illegal in most places and aren't the best solution for waste disposal. But they do work for a while so long as they are not overloaded with dish or laundry wastewater or paper.

Currently legality is a problem even when systems are not temporary. A survivor in Alaska was forced by local authorities who found out about his modest system to install an acceptably engineered, licensed, and permitted septic system at a cost exceeding $24,000!

Another option favored by some survivors is a composting toilet or an incinerating toilet. I haven't used either, but word of mouth suggests that the incinerating toilet takes lots of energy and is costly. Do your own research and see if either option could fit into your rule of threes.

We can only hope every reader who decides to retreat now will be far enough off official radars of this and other survival requirements to be able to put in a workable retreat. One requirement is valid but sometimes difficult to implement: sources of water must be at least 150 yards uphill and away from sanitary disposal. This is true even for outhouses.

In every regard, rules and regulations concerning water are calculated both to make survival impossible and to cause individuals to depend on central authorities. At their core, very few regulations have much to do with real safety and sanitation in rural areas.

Water is, of course, crucial for survivors. As mentioned, expect more and more unreasonable, controlling rules and regulations in this area.

If there is a nearby, fairly clean lake or river from which to dip, or a proven water well or spring, water may only be a passing issue for you. Perhaps the land and structure you are looking at already has an abundant water supply. Then it becomes an issue of identifying a second and a third backup source.

It is important at the outset to fully realize that these difficult issues must be addressed as soon as possible. If you are a neophyte in terms of retreating or securing water supplies, you now have at least some familiarity of your options so you can begin your own research suited to your needs.

CHAPTER FIVE

FINDING VALUE DURING THE COLLAPSE

Now we arrive at an area of survival that continues to evade me: how to know what will be valuable during a catastrophic, prolonged economic collapse. Truth be told, although I have tried mightily, I haven't figured this one out. This in spite of my having lived and worked in, as well as observed, a great number of collapsed countries, economies, and societies. Not in order of importance, these include Hungary, Rhodesia, Japan, Cuba, Italy, Greece, Cyprus, Somalia, Ireland, Portugal, Iceland, Mexico, and Spain, as well as Germany after World War II. My father also heavily briefed me on conditions he faced in Germany after World War I. My granddad on my mother's side had similar comments regarding life in the Ukraine, principally Odessa.

It seems that it would be helpful to explore the issue of what possesses universal value and retains that value during an economic collapse. In other words, what is our trading stock?

To those with real, on-the-ground, extensive experience with finding value and operating in a collapsed economy—let's communicate through Paladin (send contact information to Ragnar Benson, c/o Paladin Press, Gunbarrel Tech Center, 7077 Winchester Circle, Boulder, CO 80301). I will maintain a discussion board on this subject from which we can all profit. But please provide only actual, real experiences—not theoretical or hypothetical ones. Survival isn't about theory, as I said earlier.

Firearms and ammunition, for instance, are conventionally purported by survivors—in theory only—as excellent universal trading stock. Yet history shows that in both Germany and Rhodesia, which had extensive gun cultures, neither guns nor ammunition took on universal, or even any appreciable, extra value within these societies.

On the other hand, my father recalled trading a baby grand piano to some German farmers for several sacks of potatoes in about 1920. As a kid, he also recalled following passing horse carts on the street where he lived in hopes of scooping up some "road apple" droppings, which were traded to some gardeners for produce. How's that for an unusual, unthought-of trade item?

After World War II, shovels, rakes, hoes, axes, and even pairs of scissors, along with garden seeds, were prized trade items in recovering Germany. Though regulated, currently there is a thriving international commerce in seeds, bulbs, and cuttings. Of course, this infrastructure could fail during a prolonged crisis, in which case small, rural shops would likely pop up to produce these vitally needed products. I'm not overly optimistic about laying back garden tools as valuable trading stock today because tools are so easily produced in farm shops. Those who need them can easily make their own or have them made cheaply. On the other hand, domestic sales of surplus garden seeds might be brisk.

After living in Cuba during the 1950s, I returned there for two extensive periods in the 1990s during a time of severe privation. I observed Cubans literally begging for bars of soap, toothpaste and toothbrushes, pens, aspirin, vitamins, socks, and underwear in that precise order. Fidel would want me to note that this was during the time of their maximum distress when Cuba had been cut off financially by the Soviets. And, of course, that this stress "was the fault of the Americans!" Few of us leaving Cuba had anything left in our suitcases when we landed in Toronto.

Common wisdom suggests that collapsed economies peddle their women. I'm not clear if this is cause or effect, and some collapsed states do not seem to put their women on sale. There was little sign of hookers in today's Athens, but in Cuba and Iran prostitution is common, as it was in postwar Italy and Germany. Will this be the case in collapsed America? Time will tell.

Entrepreneurial Somalis sold Coke bottles full of gasoline and diesel for fuel at small roadside stands at absolutely ruinous prices. Spare parts for vehicles—including brake shoes, clutch plates, alternators, batteries, tires, and tubes—were in great demand. This was in spite of the fact that some of these folks were very clever at refurbishing, rebuilding, and repairing.

It's my observation that many Spaniards today seem to care less. They don't even bother to trade unless it's for cigarettes and booze. Bureaucratic employees, including police—who cannot legally be fired and cannot be paid because there is absolutely no money—quit work at noon. They quickly fill small sidewalk cafes and restaurants to overflowing, where they while away their time drinking Spanish red wine and smoking black-market cigarettes.

Where they get money for alcohol and tobacco is way beyond me. My grandfather recalled selling what he thought might be the last cigar in Odessa for an obscene amount, which may also have been worthless paper and coin. His point in this telling was that there always seemed to be lots of money for very frivolous, seemingly unimportant items.

My time in Hungary in 1959, just three years after the Hungarian revolt, tells us little to nothing about survival. Our activities and contacts were so tightly controlled by ruling Communists that we had little to no idea what Hungarian survivors were really doing or how they were doing it.

Portuguese survivors are briefly removed from their time living in a dictatorship. And they have pretty much remained an agrarian society. They were miserable and self-sufficient on small rural plots then, and they are miserable and self-sufficient now. As they say, "nothing much changes." Their lesson is obvious: while survival in the city is essentially impossible, it can be done out in the country, even by people who don't prepare adequately for it, provided retreating becomes a committed goal.

Mexico experiences collapses on an almost regular schedule. These difficult times have always been fairly temporary. Mexicans seem to rely on that optimism, and they are generally a very tough, hardscrabble folk. Based on observing two separate economic collapses in Mexico, it seems as though bar girls, waitresses, female bartenders, and prostitutes quickly pick up any economic slack. Mexicans also switch to U.S. dollars rather than pesos with lightning speed.

Survival applications from these countries for our situation? Readers should feel free to make any applicable ones for themselves.

Many astute investors, not really retreaters or survivors, hold gold bullion or coins. This is generally more as an investment hedge than as survival currency. There are many problems with assuming that gold is a good survival trade commodity. Gold may be an excellent economic hedge against inflation, but in my opinion it is a really poor survival good.

First, it generally comes in denominations too large to be a practical, day-to-day trade item. As a practical matter, this hurdle can sometimes be overcome. Trade gold for large items such as several barrels of diesel fuel, large stocks of repair parts for generators, medical services and supplies, or large quantities of food items that become your personal additional trading stock. The problem is that survivors using gold frequently have to dramatically overpay for some vital small items, and opportunities to trade are many times fewer when only large trades can be considered.

Another problem is that markets for gold may be restricted and narrow. How will you know, for instance, what gold is really worth the day of the trade? It will be worth what the other guy says it's worth, which probably isn't to your advantage.

Nevertheless, some German survivors made extensive use of gold as trading stock after their wars. Personally, I have always had serious moral reservations about gold as currency. Gold earns no interest, and, more important, gold holders are not making their surplus funds available for loans. In some societies, such as in India, this problem can become pervasive. Without money on deposit, financial institutions cannot make loans to businesses to purchase capital goods needed for production, expansion, and hiring. Within societies where gold is extensively

Finding Value During the Collapse 43

held, there is always a chronic shortage of funds at reasonable rates for entrepreneurs to purchase trucks, lathes, boats, barges, factory buildings, stamping machines, food processing machinery, storage warehouses, and such like.

Of course, this has little to do with retreating in a collapsed economy. It only explains potential financing that may have helped that economy avoid collapse.

A basic Jewish survival philosophy from ancient times teaches that the best trading stock is professional ability, which is portable and, unlike all other private possessions, cannot be confiscated. Recall that Jews have traditionally been summarily, arbitrarily, and wickedly kicked from place to place throughout their long, bitter history. But wherever they landed, they seemed to prosper. As trained doctors, accountants, dentists, nurses, lawyers, jewelers, and teachers, they were often able to quickly deploy these skills, creating a new and adequate life for themselves and their families. But this requires that survivors accurately predict which skills and talents will be in demand during an economic collapse. At this writing, it seems that midwives, butchers, and mechanics will be in demand as opposed to social workers, counselors, bureaucratic regulators, and telephone repair technicians. In Spain and Greece, for example, huge numbers of personal telephones have been disconnected, mostly for nonpayment.

This brings up a really important and difficult point. Although it is virtually impossible to predict exactly what parts, supplies, or services will become tradable in any specific location, it is vitally important that you, as a survivor, have the ability and resources to produce something real, tangible, and necessary. For instance, think fixing tires as opposed to playing a guitar, repairing chain saws instead of interpreting government edicts, or processing food rather than teaching diversity.

Think of the $2 rubber gasket needed to seal a fuel filter back into a diesel tractor engine. Up until we finally found one in our stored mechanical supplies, it looked like we would have to have a near neighbor make one from scratch. In a real survival context, what would that have been worth? Our tractor would not have run without this tiny, otherwise inexpensive part.

Successful survivors should look seriously at any and every job that comes their way. Some might discover they are gifted at a job they never considered before, while many must keep looking till they find the in-demand skill at which they can really excel. I think of some extremely able Chinese gunsmiths I encountered in East Africa in this regard. These guys were incredible! What was their background? I don't know, but I doubt that it was gunsmithing.

Certainly medical/dental skills and supplies will be in high demand. Currently throughout the entire country of Greece, there are no medical supplies and precious few doctors, nurses, or dentists. Many of Greece's medical professionals have immigrated to greener pastures in Germany, Australia, Canada, the United Kingdom, and even to many of the nearby Muslim countries. There are very few medical supplies in Greece because government officials controlled most imports and haven't paid for any medical shipments for well over a year. Virtually all medicines and supplies are imported, as very little is locally produced. Medicine and treatment are dispensed as part of government largesse. Official medical pipelines have shriveled and essentially died. A small bottle of glucosamine tablets, for instance, was priced at $75 in an Athens pharmacy.

Yet some few medical supplies and services are available—it depends how badly you want them and how much you are willing to pay. A shadowy black market has emerged. Some brave entrepreneurs have collected what cash they could and traveled to Central Europe to purchase medicines. Smuggling these into Greece isn't tough. Rural border control agents haven't been paid in months, and most aren't there to check people coming in and their cargo. The problem, of course, is receiving payment when selling these supplies. Though Greece is still on the euro, not many remain in circulation there.

Greece is very much like Cuba in that regard. During my last visit in 1996, I encountered a four-year-old girl with an easily medicated form of early epilepsy. Since she was the young daughter of nobody important and she was officially expendable, absolutely no meds were available to control the seizures destroying her tiny brain. I consider it a high point in my career that I was able to smuggle enough medications in for her so that she was properly treated till puberty, when her condition ceased.

It is a fact that medicines and medical skills have always been, and always will be, in demand in a collapsed economy. And keep in mind that medical providers are not just limited to formally trained people. I have observed old women who provided absolutely wonderful medical care—they have stitched up wounds, set broken bones, and delivered breech babies.

Stockpiling generators, repair parts, common truck and auto engine parts, light bulbs, batteries, booze, common medical supplies, long-lived garden seeds (the shelf life of garden seeds is a complex issue; consult an authoritative reference before selecting your seeds) is highly recommended at this time. Small tractor and truck engine oil filters may be in short supply during a crisis. This category of goods provides excellent value at any time but especially during an emergency. But if you're thinking of storing parts for bartering, you should reconsider. Because large numbers of types, sizes, and makes are out there, storage and inventory of replacement parts for the average guy is problematic. Unless you are an expert, any storage plan will be a hopeless hit-or-miss deal. Quickly all popular units will be gone, leaving you with expensive, nonusable junk behind. It might be best to lay back a six-year supply for your own vehicles, generators, and tractors rather than anticipating neighborhood demand.

Knowledgeable retreaters suggest doubling up on necessary retreat items. Of course, this won't work for such perishables as cereal, ice cream, and dairy products. But for sugar, salt, flour, dried peas, lentils, rice, maul handles, saw files, gloves, baking soda, flashlight bulbs, batteries, boots, glue, toilet paper, aspirin, and items that have long storage lives, this plan is mostly workable. After the crisis hits, such essential stuff as 55-gallon barrels, plastic tarps, and durable raincoats simply disappear from store shelves. Better buy them now.

The trouble with this system is that most people do not commonly stock up on these items. As a result, unless you as the retreater make a conscientious effort to anticipate what will be needed and have sufficient funds to buy them, these items will not be stockpiled. Too much will fall through the cracks.

One school of thought is to lay back as much as you can afford and anticipate for personal needs and then trade skills for what is missing later. This brings to mind a woman in East Africa who taught a one-month course for newly arrived, deeply rural women who could only get to a store once or twice a year. This was a real eye-opener for folks who never thought about how to accurately anticipate common household needs a year in advance. Even with great instruction, it took several years for new folks to really get good at this business.

We also have to believe that, in a large, desperate economy such as ours, many necessary items will continue to be manufactured. Perhaps it will be on a much smaller scale or on a regional basis at horribly inflated prices, but manufactured and marketed nevertheless. I think of Cuba, where an industry sprang up refurbishing disposable cigarette lighters by refueling and installing new flints, or Africa, where fairly serviceable shoes were made from old tires.

In rural Turkey I visited a small factory that restored and rebuilt lead acid vehicle batteries. These guys took two or three unserviceable batteries, took them apart, and assembled one fairly good one from the still functional parts. Eventually all these batteries were used up, but in the interim of perhaps three or four years, vehicle owners did not have to buy new imported batteries, which were horribly expensive. Preppers in this country have been doing this for about a generation. Read the classifieds in *Mother Earth News* for all the supplies you'd ever want for rebuilding lead-acid batteries. They are even for sale designed to be rebuilt, or you can buy plans to build them from scratch.

I have also encountered entrepreneurs who reused engine oil

filters using rolls of toilet paper as new filter material. This was extremely labor intensive and certainly only stopgap, but a procedure that was workable. It also illustrates my observation that successful survival requires 14-hour workdays. Those used to 9-to-5 jobs and pensions just won't cut it. This perhaps explains what we see in France and Spain, where real productive work has been scarce for years.

Immediately prior to the conclusion of World War II, the economies of occupied Jersey and Guernsey collapsed. Jersey and Guernsey are two unique self-governing island nations of the United Kingdom that the Germans occupied during the war. Few people on the islands actually starved, but pervasive, desperate hunger swept through both German occupiers and the residents. Is the lesson here that food is a great trade item?

Perhaps in some circumstances, trading food to city people might be workable, but recall we are purposefully locating in rural areas where abundant food is produced. Food might be sufficiently bountiful to trade. Keep in mind, however, that your retreat may be compromised by trade with outsiders and trade with locals won't be needed. Also keep in mind that almost every famine in the last 100 years has been caused by governments, often intentionally. Think of past famines in China, Russia, Ukraine, Cuba, India, Somalia, and other countries around the globe. Retreaters may incur their wrath by making food available.

As mentioned, I have not observed guns and ammo being useful trade items in any of the 14 collapsed economies with which I have been personally involved. The closest would be in current Greece, where a very small market has developed for personal firearms for city people who are unable to move to the country.

This might come as a horrible shock to theoretical survival thinkers who also tend to be admitted "gun nuts." There is nothing wrong with being a gun enthusiast, having sufficient ammunition laid back, and being willing and able to defend your family. Yet successful survivors will not rely solely on hunting for their food, and there are much better ways of defending a retreat than shooting it out. Besides, in deep rural areas, theft usually isn't a pervasive problem.

For instance, I secure all of our year's meat with only two rounds for my rifle. Keeping marauding birds away from our orchards requires another half box of .22s, and I occasionally expend a rifle round or two controlling wolves. It doesn't take much stored ammo or reloading supplies for me to satisfy this level of yearly demand. This may seem dangerously low to some of you. Point taken. You should store what you think your family will need, but keep in mind that it takes much less ammunition to survive than most people imagine.

This leaves us with lessons from Japan. I haven't included Japan in my previous examples, mostly because there are few if any survival lessons to be learned from a culture that just cannot change. Japanese people are incredibly accepting of their circumstances, no matter how awful. They continue to live with massive overregulation, horribly intrusive permit requirements, senseless environmental goals, an all-powerful government spying on their every movement, tremendously expensive import requirements, and crony politicians living high at the expense of average citizens. The economy subsides, groans, and dies, but almost no Japanese see any reason to change it or to personally make things better for themselves. They just grind on and on, calmly accepting whatever comes their way.

Perhaps there is a lesson after all. We as surviving retreaters see the vast majority of our friends, families, and acquaintances as optimistically accepting of the inevitable, just like the Japanese, continually hoping that things don't get any worse. A few of us will retreat, trusting that we can survive until our economy heals itself and we can start over again. Not many but a few.

With that, we leave the issue of value in a collapsed economy. I repeat again: absolutely anyone with actual, real-life—not theoretical—expertise in a collapsed country or society, please contact me. I travel most of the year, so contacts are best made through Paladin. No doubt we might share some extremely interesting information.

CHAPTER SIX

THREE SOURCES OF FOOD

Planning for three valid, workable, entirely independent food sources will be much different now than it would have been under what we might term "conventional" survival. Past survivors assumed they could store enough food to see them through the crisis, with minimal scrounging and resupply. Most today know that is not true. They know that they must be able to resupply their food stores, acquired from third-party sources (through purchase or trade) and self-production.

Resupply under this new reality won't be easy. Conventionally, we supposed an emergency would pass in months or a couple of years at most. Knowledgeable sources—based on what's happening in Cuba, Greece, Italy, Spain, Ireland, and many other struggling nations—predict that our problems will last four or five years at a minimum, with some predicting up to 10 years. A two-year survival horizon is hopelessly optimistic.

Don't get me wrong: adequate storage against lean times is still very important, but working out means of resupply is much more important. Resupply will come in herky-jerky fits and starts. Going to the supermarket even once every three months will be a distant memory only. Planning ahead and then seizing any opportunities that arise will be vital.

With the exception of Russia during the late 1920s and early '30s, where peasant farmers were intentionally starved to death, and of the Ukraine up until modern times, where lack of seeds, fertilizers, pesticides, storage facilities, and work ethic vital to any efficient agricultural enterprise precluded adequate farm production, all collapsed economies continued to produce some food. This was true even in Cuba, our worst-case example of a collapsed economy. My point is that all mass starvations worldwide during the last 100 years were caused by hostile governments. As examples, think of Russia and of China during Mao's Cultural Revolution in the 1950s. The Ukraine once had an historic reputation as a breadbasket but, because of government policy, never progressed into an era of modern, high-yield agricultural production.

Predicting future government food policy in the United States is hopelessly difficult, yet you can be reasonably certain that a woefully inadequate supply of food will find its way into larger cities and it may become very expensive even out in the rural areas. But some food will always be produced. Knowing where to look for it and how to secure it are the challenges.

Great production problems persist. City people often fail to realize the extent modern technology plays in the delivery of an increased abundance of food. Our large surplus of food results from continually improved seed varieties and pesticides. These new varieties increasingly resist weeds, require less water, and make better use of modern fertilizers and pesticides while dramatically increasing yields. Today's farmers calculate that current varieties of seed for corn, wheat, barley, edible beans, peas, lentils, and soybeans last only about five years. After that, new improved varieties emerge and are planted by commercial farmers. Old varieties pass, never to be heard of again.

It seems extremely unlikely that many new varieties of seeds or pesticides will be available in the collapsed economy we see ahead. Technology for needed improvements won't disappear, but it will definitely go into hibernation for several years. As a result, diseases and insects will decimate our crops, leading to materially decreased harvests that otherwise could be sent into cities or used as feed grains. As a matter of policy, some politically well-connected environmental groups strongly oppose modern agricultural production. Ultimate victory for these special interest groups is impossible to predict, but so far they have been far more successful than we might have initially supposed.

Rural people in Germany and Poland after World Wars I and II quickly had some crops in the ground. They may have been relatively low-yield garden or truck crops, but survivors in the country knew they had to get something edible growing as soon as possible. Food production in southern latitudes, where growing seasons are longer, was a bit easier. Pity a starving farmer's wife in north Germany or Poland who, when hostilities finally passed, also tragically had to face the fact that it was too late in the season to successfully grow anything edible.

Commercial agricultural production notwithstanding, 21st-century survivors are almost certainly going to have to learn how to garden in the area in which they choose to retreat. A very few especially talented survivors *may* be able to trade skills for all their food in rural areas. Yet, as a general rule, they are going to have to assume they will have to produce at least some of their own food. You may be able to go to local farmers for some basic food that will sustain life as one of the three food-supply sources, and stored food supplies will still be important. But self-production will also be vital.

Even experienced gardeners find that reliably raising vegetables in a different environment involves trial and error. Crops that flourish in a humid, temperate climate might well fail in an arid or alpine region. Your best bet is to retreat with local friends or relatives who already know how to garden locally, or to find friendly neighbors willing to provide accurate advice on the best crops and methods for your new area. There are excellent gardening references available for every region. You should use these to do your research before your life depends on the crops you grow.

Living entirely on wild edibles is probably not a viable option, at least until retreaters learn the local bounty. Plus, in a catastrophic meltdown, great numbers of people may be out foraging for the same limited supply. In which case, common cattails, acorns, and other wild edibles will quickly disappear.

Some years ago, a few scornful reporters picked me up at what was then called National Airport (it has since been renamed

Ronald Reagan National Airport) in Washington, D.C. As we headed into the city, they began to interview me for a story on survival for the mainstream media. One ignorantly stated that no wild edibles could be harvested in or near large cities. Like a pouncing leopard, I pointed out that we were driving past some very large beds of cattails that—when properly harvested—yielded flower heads that could be roasted, green shoots that made nutritious steamed vegetables, pollen that substituted wonderfully for wheat flour, and roots that—even in winter—provided a filling though not very tasty or nutritious gruel, much like watery mashed potatoes. Yes, they grudgingly conceded, but how long will those beds of cattails last in cities with millions of hungry residents? Maybe longer than one might suppose, I replied, because few city people knew about these wild edibles and many refused to work hard enough to harvest them, much less endure their foreign, often very different, taste.

Continuing, we drove on through a nice oak tree–lined boulevard into a large park, where acorns covered the ground. "With lots of hard work harvesting and preparing them, acorns are another excellent source of food," I quickly pointed out.

This time one of the smarter reporters was ready for me. "Yes, but acorns are poisonous, aren't they?"

To a varying degree they are, I acknowledged, but knowledgeable survivors know to wash tannic acid out of the meat of common acorns, creating good, nutritious food. Their point—actually quite a good one—was that unless retreaters know what they are doing with wild edibles, they are likely to quickly kill or sicken themselves and their families with harvested foods they know little about. And, of course, most common varieties of this stuff will quickly disappear even in very rural areas.

On the other hand, today's retreaters cannot assume such ignorance on the part of their neighbors. Most retreaters are knowledgeable, highly motivated people, who if they don't know about cattails and acorns in the first place will make it their first order of business to find out. Thus, local supplies of edibles will be harvested quickly, and retreaters will know enough not to eat the inedible parts of plants. Wild edibles have provided vital sustenance to great numbers of survivors in times past, principally because governments that want to pacify angry city people who expect to be taken care of will confiscate conventional food from rural people to send to cities. But governments have a tough time confiscating wild edibles.

Think that can't happen in the United States? During Hurricane Katrina, local farmers reported that the Federal Emergency Management Agency (FEMA) conducted an inventory of local farms and what they produced. Why did FEMA make this food assessment, and what was its intention? Who knows, but it made some area farmers very uneasy. Plus, you don't want to advertise the contents of your survival pantry to anyone living nearby or passing through who might be running low on food and who might be unscrupulous (or desperate) enough to try to force you to share yours.

Therefore, retreaters operating under this new, modern reality are going to have to be very cautious about revealing the source and location of any food items they may be relying on. This would include gardens, as well as freezers and cellars stocked with prepared foods.

During our past financial crises, survivalists assumed that they could live on wild game trapped from surrounding fields and forests. Today this is less feasible. In part to discourage sport hunting, some powerful environmental groups have supported reintroduction of a super-large species of wolf into many of our remote and not-so-remote rural areas. This is especially true in northern areas of the United States that have large tracts of sparsely populated ground, which is exactly the area to which many retreaters will look.

These large, hungry predators have expanded their populations dramatically and are impossible to control using traditional hunting and trapping methods. As a result, deer, elk, and bear populations on which survivors intended to rely on for food have disappeared. One mountain retreater reports an area that traditionally supported 50-plus resident deer, a smaller group of elk, and the occasional bear now has only three or four deer, no elk, and no bears. The rest were killed—some eaten—by wolves. Because of especially loathsome parasites they carry, we do not plan to eat wolf, should we be so fortunate to catch one. Edible wild dogs have been numerous, but perhaps wolves will get these as well.

Some wild game may still persist in your rural area of choice. Learning to trap or snare them is less difficult than learning to successfully hunt, which is never wise in a survival context. Labor-intensive sport hunting is seldom wise in a survival situation, as more energy may be invested than is earned.

Collecting smaller wild game not affected by wolves—such as raccoons, rabbits, possums, turkeys, quail, muskrats, common rats, cats, and dogs, and similar creatures that can avoid wolves or outbreed them—might still be possible. Retreaters are advised not to overlook semi-wild game. I think, for example, of my father and his brothers who crept into night-darkened churches and train terminals where they perilously climbed up to snatch unsuspecting barn pigeons from their roosts. (There are still dovecotes in the ancient Edomite fortress of Masada. King Herod, who built the fortress, evidently planned that his pigeons—which produced two plump young ones every 40 days while scaring up their own food and water—should provide an occasional protein meal.)

Don't forget about waterborne sources of food, including fish and turtles that are relatively easily trapped. Turtles provided an excellent source of protein for us back on the farm when we were very poor. A basic, absolute rule of food survival is that you must always eat whatever is available . . . with thanks.

Contrast the attitude of the Chinese with those of the Indians in this regard. Indians from the subcontinent have huge numbers of food prejudices and beliefs. Some won't eat pork, some eschew beef, some avoid seafood, and still others abstain from meat of any kind. As a result, they frequently starve or are extremely hungry, all voluntarily. The Chinese eat virtually anything if it is prepared properly, including snakes, sea slugs, and birds' nests. They even convince themselves that these are delicacies! Hunger and starvation exist in China, but only as a result of government edict, not religious or personal conviction, and not in recent years.

This brings up another important point for retreaters putting together their own private three-part food security program. Many successful retreaters will probably be as well off keeping rabbits, chickens, ducks, goats, or geese as they would trying to learn to catch wild game. Only a small amount of ground is sufficient to provide feed for small livestock, especially if you supplement their diet with garden scraps, such as corn stalks or veggies that have gone to seed. Goats, especially, are easy to keep. They live on virtually nothing, eating mostly weeds, some of which are too prickly to pull with bare hands. Goats are an excellent source of red meat and dairy, as well as fiber. Learning curves for raising goats and other small domestic livestock are short and gentle. Yet unless survivors know how to butcher the livestock, this is another nonstarter.

Retreaters who currently don't know how to slaughter, butcher, and process both wild and domestic animals *might* be able to rely on someone who does, but why take the chance? Butchering meat is not rocket science; anyone can learn. You are much better off doing this job yourself. You may not like this work, but learning how to do it takes only a time or two.

Given a few years to practice, raising and processing small domestic livestock can be learned. A possibly more difficult job for a new outsider will be learning how to get along and trade with farmers. Condescension won't work. Acting like a farmer won't work. Trying to impress locals with money, good looks, or importance certainly won't work. Getting to know them well before an emergency and trying very hard to listen and genuinely see things from their point of view might possibly work. Providing a valuable service almost always works.

Dealing with farmers you know is an extremely important skill. Recall that you settled in an agricultural area where an abundance of food is grown and stored for a reason. Unless this means of resupply is available, there is little chance of lasting four to six years.

Farmers in your retreat area may raise chickens, ducks, hogs, cattle, sheep, goats, or even catfish. Livestock farmers always have a small percentage of crippled, downer, or damaged livestock that cannot be sent to conventional markets. Properly handled and processed, these will make good eating for you and your family. The trick will be getting these farmers to sell you their culls or perhaps some of their regular production before shipment to market. All can be taken in, processed, and placed in a freezer for future use.

Other than butchering, food processing required for storage is another must-have skill for retreaters. This refers to "putting up" production from the garden and perhaps includes some wild edibles. Means of preserving this produce include canning, freezing, and drying. My wife and I plan to vacuum-can very little of our food production for several reasons. At harvest, edibles mature and start to spoil at a fantastically high rate and must be preserved right away. Canning, as opposed to freezing, is extremely labor intense and time consuming, requiring large amounts of scarce fuel. Additionally, canning meat and vegetables improperly can lead to poison in the jar. As a result, we currently plan to freeze almost everything.

Planting an orchard at your retreat may be an option if fruit trees prosper in the area. Just remember that it takes about four years for orchard trees to start bearing. Or perhaps an orchard already exists at your retreat, which might be another retreater's food option. Make plans to secure your harvest for preservation or bartering before it disappears from your orchard.

By the same token, scrounging or field gleaning may be another good food-replacement opportunity for you, but only if you are on good terms with local farmers and have their permission. Most city people are truly shocked when they see how much good food falls between sorting chains back onto the fields during mechanical harvest. But, of course, this is only possible if you have selected an area where tomatoes, squash, beans, and other vegetables are grown as crops. You *did* relocate to such an area, didn't you?

My guess is that most retreaters will end up in rural areas where feed grains are grown and stored rather than produce and truck crops. Field corn, wheat, barley, and soybeans are edible and life supporting, but I find them unappetizing when used right from the field storage. Soybeans from farm fields are an example. They can be roasted and ground, or they can be pressed for oil.

Raw field corn, wheat, and barley can be ground up for meal/flour and used in cakes, breads, etc., but first, the dirt clods, insect bodies, weed seeds, and straw must be sorted from field-run grains. Handling field-run feed grains can be extremely labor intensive. Yet, these items will probably be a major source of re-supply for many survivors. Also do not underestimate problems storing field-run grains and pulses. Unless thoroughly cleaned and dried to acceptable levels and then kept bone dry and cool, bugs and vermin will quickly emerge, destroying the whole lot. Farmers aerate and dry their stored grains, as well as chemically fumigate regularly.

This illustrates why laying back commercially processed and cleaned, store-bought 50-pound sacks of processed flour, dried beans, peanuts, lentils, split peas, sugar, and salt in large, sealed plastic garbage cans is wise. As long as this stuff stays reasonably cool and dry, it will remain in good shape for years (check a reliable chart for the shelf life of dried foods). But, of course, the expense of purchasing these commodities is always an issue.

Learning curves for most city people far removed from any country living experience will be steep. The problems associated with successfully picking three workable food sources and mastering them for your specific area will be tough. Perhaps substituting large amounts of cash for knowledge might work for a while. But it is always my assumption that cash is not readily available.

Currently some country-living magazines depict country life as an easy, fun, carefree, romantic, even idyllic existence. The opposite is often true for newcomers. If you are considering a rural retreat, prepare now for long hours of hard, often frustrating work . . . and some growing pains until you learn the ropes.

CHAPTER SEVEN

ENERGY

Unless individual retreaters are extremely fortunate, wise, or wealthy, providing energy during their retreat will be a very tough nut to crack. Formulating a three-part energy plan for the 21st century ranges from almost impossible to extremely difficult. Most survivors will fail, but this is no excuse for neglecting to plan now.

There are several reasons for this, most having to do with long time spans. We survivors must now look forward to—and plan for—troubling trends within our national energy industry, as well as the harsh truth that having just one form of energy will probably not be workable. In other words, electrical energy is great for light, pumping water, running freezers, and powering small tools vital to survival. But electrical energy is not so hot (pun intended) when deployed to power vehicles, including small tractors, or to warm the retreat, heat water, and cook food. Of course, electricity can be made to perform these tasks, but not without expensive, uncertain, inefficient conversions from other forms of energy. And other than in the form of diesel, firewood, and propane, energy is often tough to store. Propane may be impossible to resupply in a prolonged crisis.

Political trends may push us off the electric grid much faster than we ever would have supposed, or prices may skyrocket to the point that it is obvious that we should find other alternatives. Retreaters with extremely fat checkbooks will be able to implement work-around strategies. Yet, as in the past, I must assume most of us do not have virtually unlimited funds. Just taking advantage of regular, natural sources of energy—firewood, for example—will be costly enough. Assuming you can jump the next step to extremely costly is not realistic. In times past we assumed, wished, hoped—you pick the appropriate verb—that we could replace our energy needs by going out into surrounding fields and forests. That still might be possible for cooking and heating requirements.

A close friend carefully calculated and analyzed annual tree growth on his 15-acre woodlot and concluded that his trees will sufficiently bulk each year to exactly equal his house heating and cooking requirements. Some areas produce firewood much faster than others. Wise retreaters take this into consideration when evaluating an area for a retreat. Climate, rainfall, and soil fertility are contributing factors in annual growth rates.

You should also know that heat quality among tree species varies dramatically. Specific charts, graphs, and lists pointing to those species that are good to excellent, as well as to those that are a waste of harvesters' time, are already available in various survival manuals as well as on the Internet (just Google "wood heating"), so there is no sense replowing that ground.

Commonly, neophyte retreaters ask about using small steam engines to turn their retreat generator. To me the problems with steam engines seem insurmountable. Any wood-fired steam engine large enough to reliably crank a generator under load will be large, expensive, dirty, smelly, and clunky. Using it will require constant attention. Plus, there are very few small commercial wood-fired steam engines on the market. Steam engines are extremely fuel inefficient. Most folks are better served just burning wood in their stoves, even though most woodstoves are not terribly fuel efficient. Some are better than others, however. Study and evaluation in this area are necessary.

Wood chips, bark, sawdust, and even alternative fuels such as dried corn and animal dung may be available in some rural areas. You should not discount these alternative energy sources until you have done proper inquiry and experimentation. Other more realistic, conventional methods may be out there. In some areas retreaters may be able to access and harvest from small

Energy

seams of coal exposed in road cuts or even outcroppings on the land. Is drilling a geothermal well possible? Before laughing this thought away, inquire. Geothermal is reasonably possible in some areas of the United States.

Another very prudent retreater has access to natural gas through an abandoned mill in his area. That's good as long as it lasts, but caution is required. Gas supplies could be cut off at any time, necessitating that this must not be the fellow's only source of energy.

Perhaps it hasn't been done yet, but some desperate but smart retreaters might be able to find ways of using oil shale or tar sands scrounged up in their area.

Dried peat is used in Scotland to heat houses and to power cook stoves. Harvesting, drying, storing, and using it would be horribly time consuming and back breaking, but it is clean-burning and efficient as a fuel. Many peat beds are scattered about the United States; in fact, there are an estimated 80 million acres of deposit in the continental United States. It could be an option if you live near a bog or local source and wood or coal is unavailable or too expensive.

In another instance, a retreater put a generator behind a small, low dam in a stream near his retreat. He reports the miserable contraption requires constant attention, as well as costly maintenance but does recharge his wet cell batteries sufficiently to power his freezer and lights and some water pumps. However, it is insufficient for room heaters, water heaters, and ranges, which require way too much electrical power to be practical. And, he reports, his system was very expensive to install and could run afoul of regulators who don't want private people to take advantage of what they claim is public water, no matter how insignificant the amount used.

We used a large home-built windmill in remote East Africa to power our air compressors, some fans, a few lights, a sewing machine, radios, and some small water pumps. Sufficient power was stored in a large bank of batteries to get us minimally by during times when the wind did not blow. Our system profited by being in a place high on a mountain outcrop, where winds were fairly consistent. It was, however, very expensive—almost $25,000—even though we designed and built it ourselves. And it required constant maintenance and supervision. This is another reminder that retreaters with lots of money will probably come closer than the rest of us to implementing a valid energy rule of threes.

Any discussion of ruinously expensive energy sources brings us to solar. True enough, solar panels have both fallen in price and increased in efficiency in recent years. But the high cost of these systems is not found in the solar panels themselves, but rather in batteries, inverters, switches, copper wire, junction boxes, and other parts required to assemble a reliable system. The last solar system with which I was involved that was sufficiently large to run an entire retreat cost about $65,000, and only about $8,000 of that was for solar panels! And this was before the price of copper went out of sight.

Solar could nicely cover a portion of a retreater's electrical needs if he can stand the tariff and lived in a place conducive to solar power production. Just remember that the rule of thumb is that solar panels produce about 17 percent of their rated daily capacity.

Most retreaters I know will probably rely on firewood and diesel fuel for their energy requirements: firewood to heat and cook, and diesel to run generators and provide some minimal transportation and hauling.

Let's take firewood first. It will be immediately incumbent on new retreaters to figure out which species of trees found in their area provide the best heat. Then they will have to figure out how to safely and economically run a chain saw necessary for wood harvesting. Certainly in times past a great deal of firewood was harvested with hand axes and saws, but most modern folks no longer have that much time or energy.

Operating a chain saw requires that you learn how to service, repair, and maintain the saws. This would include learning to properly sharpen the saw's chains. Finding a local expert in rural areas to help with these duties is usually not difficult, but chain saws require constant hour-by-hour adjustment and servicing best done by knowledgeable owner/users.

Recently in a small rural community where logging was still a main industry, I asked about purchasing a replacement chain for a worn one on my saw. "Is it a Stihl or Husqvarna?" a helpful local asked, hitting the main issue head on. Universally, industry experts claim that any other brands of saw are basically unusable junk requiring far too much time and maintenance. And often these inferior saws won't do the work. Neophyte chain saw buyers beware! This illustrates once again the importance of building up a small supply of replacement parts for their chain saws and other tools.

Using a chain saw requires ongoing access to several gallons of gasoline, plus a quart of two-cycle oil and a gallon of bar oil per year. Unlike gasoline, the oil products can be stored long term.

As mentioned, more than just firewood is utilized in stoves, including anything that burns. Many retreaters hereabouts roll old newspapers into five-inch fire logs. Feeding these into stoves, along with a few sticks of good oak or cherry, cuts our wood consumption by about 10 percent, which is meaningful anytime but especially during a survival situation. Burning paper also increases the amount of ash, which makes excellent fertilizer for our garden. Make sure you have a good supply of old papers because newspapers may become more scarce during the crisis, or you may be unable to continue your subscription.

Many rural retreaters plan to use diesel fuel to power their small tractors and generators. Number two diesel has about 20 percent more energy per gallon than standard gasoline. Diesel fuel is easier to store and will probably be used in vehicles at and about your retreat. Red diesel number two fuel oil is off-the-road fuel. Sold tax-free, it often costs less than gasoline. City people, unaccustomed to using diesel fuel, seldom know about inexpensive, tax-free red diesel fuel. It is red to discourage diesel car and truck owners from using this cheap fuel on highways (more on this subject in subsequent chapters).

Ready for some good news? Absolutely every country and

society suffering from a collapsed economy continued to have at least some fuel available. In our worst example, Cuba, gasoline and diesel were tightly rationed so that only tourists paying exorbitant prices could afford them. Farming was undertaken entirely with horses and oxen. There were no private cars on the road and few government ones either. Prices for fuel in Iceland and Greece were always up in the nosebleed section of the price range, and they still are. But fuel is still available

Farmers in the United States will certainly have access to some diesel fuel. Little to no gasoline is used in modern farm tractors and other machinery, so gasoline could be a problem even if very little is required. Use of precious supplies of gasoline for chain saws will be miniscule. Some large farmers have diesel-storage capacities in tens of thousands of gallons on their farms, so buying some fuel from them to top off your supply may be possible. In many cases, this will be your best (if not only) means of resupply late in the crisis. There is no way to predict future prices or supplies down on the farm.

Those living near our borders might be able to cross into Mexico or Canada to purchase supplies of fuel, but this assumes that Canada and Mexico will have ample supplies. Both countries produce lots of energy, but I'm not sure I would count on either as a source of affordable fuel in a survival situation.

Without fuel, city people with all their attendant problems will mostly remain in the cities. Think of the evacuation of New Orleans during Katrina in this regard! The only exception will be retreaters who, like European Jews in the 1930s, waited too long to leave and then had to depart in a mad rush. On the other hand, lack of fuel may contribute materially to peace and order out in the country, as few will actually make it out into rural areas.

Farmers and ranchers will have necessary pumps, funnels, hoses, barrel taps, and other tools with which to access their stored fuel supplies. An excellent question then becomes how will you, the new retreater, get this fuel home, store it, and then access it in time of need? Assuming, of course, that your relationship with farmers will even allow you to purchase fuel from them.

Economics, forced and applied, will cut energy usage at most retreats. Think of hand pumps on wells, hand digging gardens, and solar-heated bags of shower water among many others in this regard.

As if all of this is not sufficiently challenging, a number of very powerful forces currently work against any kind of energy-supply program we retreaters may try to implement. Some of these may make life even more difficult for all of us. Dramatic new oil patch technology, for instance, is currently enabling the United States to again be energy self-sufficient. Rather than celebrating these remarkable new supplies, the Sierra Club, one among many protesters, has vowed to do its best to shut down all this oil and gas production. Coal production, which currently provides 40 percent of our electricity, is under constant attack by multiple environmental organizations. We may all be involuntarily disconnected from the grid sooner than we suspect. What will city people, who have made no provision to provide for themselves, do then?

It doesn't take a Phi Beta Kappa to realize we indeed live in perilous, difficult, and interesting times.

CHAPTER EIGHT

SHELTER

Effective planning for shelter in a 21st-century context is complex but, unlike some other elements of retreating, is fairly straightforward. You might even use the term *doable*, especially over medium- to long-term planning horizons.

Much of this boils down to the fact that you've got to shelter *someplace*, and it might as well be a place that provides some hope for the future. Choose a location that includes security, obscurity, and sufficient resources for effectively going on with your life.

"Do I really, truly need to apply the rule of threes to my survival shelter program?" is probably the first question that pops into most people's minds. This is certainly an issue that can profit from careful thought and evaluation.

The reason for backup plans B and C for food, water, energy, and other survival necessities addresses the eternal reality that these few items are absolutely vital yet finite and may not be available in life-or-death emergencies. In other words, it is impossible for mere mortals to accurately know future events. But it is comparatively easy to preplan now for alternate means of obtaining vital requirements when faced with catastrophic, unforeseen future events. The same is essentially true for shelter. And planning shelter backup plans, especially compared to other elements, is relatively straightforward, easy, and inexpensive.

If you can set aside the actions of hostile governments and citizens of the type that severely impacted the lives of people in Nazi Germany, Soviet Ukraine, and Cuba, believing this could not possibly happen in the United States (which many survivors believe is not only possible but indeed likely), the next greatest danger out in the country is from natural disasters. Could an earthquake, fire, landslide, flood, drought, tornado, or other calamity wipe out your primary retreat? This quickly becomes the question.

What to do then? Obviously in most places in the United States, human life without shelter cannot go on for long. Do we wait for government help, realizing from past disasters how ineffective that really is? In a financially corrupt, monumentally broke, collapsed economy, this may be a very long wait. This may not be a perfect example, but recall all those folks in the aftermath of Hurricane Katrina along the Gulf Coast, coupled to half-hearted, ineffective government relief efforts. Or more recently, Tropical Storm Sandy in the mid-Atlantic and northeastern states, especially New York and New Jersey. It is better to have a plan B and a plan C.

An extremely basic yet important rule of survival is to *never* let yourself become a refugee. Fleeing to an unknown place and relying on strangers for hoper-groper benevolence is a surefire recipe for disaster.

During times of relatively sparse populations (with no more than 2.5 million natives living out on the land), it was possible to head out into open places carrying along a sack of dried beans, mess kit, rifle, blanket, ax, and canteen. By shooting a few rabbits or quail, you could eke out an existence for years at a time. This is no longer true in any place in this world of which I am personally aware.

Historical records outlining mistreatment and abuse of refugees are indisputable: they become someone else's property to do with as that person or organization dictates. Based on experiences of at least 100 years, the treatment of refugees during an extended and serious economic collapse won't be good. Only a fortunate few will actually survive . . . with an emphasis on "fortunate few."

Because of the very long duration retreaters must plan for, and because alternatives are universally bad, there must be a shelter plan that takes a survivor and his family to a safe place where adequate preparations have already been made to live. The importance of this concept is impossible to overemphasize.

While your shelter plan itself may be straightforward, the methods of accessing the retreat in an emergency could get messy. Your place of refuge must be easily and quickly accessible if, in fact, you are not already living there permanently. As stressed over and over, moving to a remote, obscure, rural location is your best option for securing your family's survival. However, combining ease of access with vital obscurity is often very difficult but correspondingly important.

The danger of natural disasters may seem very remote and issues of overpopulation and obscurity might have already been settled, so why worry about planning for three separate survival shelters? Other factors play a part, including the fact that planning a three-part program is often quick and easy. Given a bit of thought, there is often little debate.

Many, if not most, American families, for example, could quickly, easily, and logically use a travel camper or another mobile vehicle as their shelter plan B. Tens of millions of camper vans, pickup truck shells, and trailers are currently available in this country. Most are little used, as well as being very comfortable, and are available at affordable prices. While certainly a good, logical, and easy plan B, it may not be the best one for your family.

Retreaters will probably find that a much better, but not necessarily easier, Plan B is a barn. Barns or some sort of remodeled or purpose-built outbuildings are wonderful not only as a second emergency shelter but also as a place to store survival food, tools, implements, oil, fuel, seeds, chemicals, spare parts, and other bulky, smelly, yet essential general supplies. Fortunately many, if not most, older rural farmsteads have outbuildings that could be made to accommodate storage and shelter. Farm consolidation in just the last 30 years created thousands of these now-moldering, unused farmsteads.

Of course, many buildings on these vintage, weed-covered sites are pretty old and ratty. Worn roofs may have allowed deterioration of roof and wall joists. Depending entirely on age and current condition, cleaning and repair tasks may be daunting. Yet over a period of years—if we have that long before the SHTF—average retreaters could create serviceable buildings out of these old structures using little more than their own labor and scrounged materials. This is also true for abandoned farmhouses. Recycling old farm sites might keep you out of the greedy clutches of local planning and zoning commissions. This is another issue where you need to seek early clarification.

The only problem is that the barn or outbuilding is stationary and therefore subject to wind, fire, earthquake, or other disasters, just like your main shelter. As an alternative or additional shelter, you might consider a travel camper. Many travel campers are sufficiently mobile so that they can be moved out of harm's way or stored in an alternate, protected location. Travel campers can also be used for some storage.

A third (or even fourth) backup shelter could be an old-fashioned storm cellar, root cellar, or large cold weather tent with proper wood-fired tent stove. Since their barns are vulnerable and providing additional backup systems is cheap and easy in our current society, many smart, ambitious retreaters actively plan four or five different shelter methods: the main shelter, travel camper of some sort, barn or outbuilding, storm or root cellar, and/or a tent.

Living in tents and travel campers over long periods might present one small problem for retreaters: in some areas doing so is illegal. Our wonderful, helpful government may use these rules as a means of harassing self-sufficient retreaters.

Shelter obscurity and retreat defense are entwined. Not only because of onerous local rules regarding living in travel campers or tents, effective retreaters must be extremely cautious about being cautious. Long rural lanes at the end of obscure roads offer many advantages when siting your shelter. Recall, however, that if you are not already living there, getting to your shelter in an emergency has to be reasonably easy and planned far ahead. (I delve into this much more in the chapter on retreat security.)

As a bonus, rural shelters could provide a means of employment for rural retreaters. This may or may not be a big issue for you. Barns or rural shelters are ideal locations for automotive shops, general workshops, and food processing areas. Some may be suitable for supporting new lines of work in which survivors engage, in addition to adequately providing access to and implementing your rule-of-three provision for shelter.

In the best scenario, successful retreaters will arrange to move to rural areas or small rural villages with relatives or close friends with ample planning. In other cases, necessity will require that some of these friends will not be very close and there is little or no warning that they retreaters are coming. We know this is what happened in Germany and Poland after World War II and in Spain after its civil war. Many rural people found visitors on their doorsteps that they only vaguely knew and certainly never planned for—all of them with heart-rending stories of gross privation. This is now going on big time in Greece, Spain, and Portugal.

If you can move in with rural people, this is extremely fortuitous for you. They probably already know a thing or two about gardening, getting along with farmer friends, finding resupply sources for food and energy, and living on available water sources, as well as the likelihood of devastating natural disasters in the area and how to avoid or survive them. Yet consider the account of a hapless native of rural Georgia who had his mobile home drowned out by a hundred-year flood. Using insurance money, he replaced his mobile home and elevated it four feet above the highest previous high-water mark. Assuming that hundred-year floods occurred only every hundred years, he let his flood insurance lapse. Three years later, however, another flood put a foot and a half of water in the bottom of his new home, completely destroying it.

The moral to this true account? A second opinion regarding hazards and possible problems with life in your new region is wise.

Retreaters fortunate enough to find kindred souls already living in rural areas with whom they can relocate are probably not only fortunate but among the very few. Keys to compatibility might be those bringing needed skills, enthusiastic labor, or lots of money to the bargain. Will existing structures be adequate? Perhaps additions and adjustments could be made, sweetening the deal for existing owners.

Deciding what to do with desperate people with no usable skills, plans, money, or labor potential who just show up is much more difficult in reality than in theory. We may speculate that we would simply run them off, but when the time comes, it may not be that simple. If nothing else, for some reason or another, they may complain to authorities or otherwise create problems for you. This is another excellent reason for keeping your retreat location as isolated and secret as possible.

Other than backup shelter plans B and C, primary retreat shelters should be made as water, food, and fuel efficient as humanly possible. As just one example, proper insulation needed to economize on energy comes to mind. There are also issues of proper food storage to prevent spoilage. Controlling rats, mice, and insects is a must, as is exposure to extreme heat or cold, rain, snow, or other weather elements. Water conservation may be implemented by spreading wash and household water (gray water) on the garden.

Shelters should be stocked with work clothes, jackets, boots, belts, gloves, sweaters, shoes, and whatever else is appropriate at the retreat for all seasons. All these are easily available to retreaters before a crisis hits.

Serious retreaters universally seem to economize at their retreats. Historically, we find that much less space is used by far more people to live, cook, sleep, and eat during emergencies. Heating in winter is kept to a bare minimum, while cooling is just a pleasant dream from a bygone era. There always seem to be far more people at a retreat than originally planned. This is not all bad if the extra people are workers rather than drones. Even unskilled but anxious, energetic laborers can be a plus.

One pseudo-survival writer with no obvious real-life experience wrote that in her retreat children would be kept entertained and busy playing video games! Such unadulterated, impractical bull-puckery (a term I seldom use) is impossible to imagine in a real-life, true retreat situation.

If the retreat is to survive as a working unit, I can absolutely guarantee that even six- or eight-year-olds, in addition to being homeschooled, will be hauling wood and water, helping with food preparation, harvesting and preserving crops, washing dishes and clothes, refueling machines, and performing other vital retreat tasks. It's going to have to be like current Third World situations, where children have many heavy chores from a very early age, perhaps as young as four.

What do you do if someone shows up with small kids in tow? It is valid to ask about their skills, work ethic, and personal discipline. The parents don't like these questions? Then they have no place in your retreat shelter. This sounds cruel, but retreating is not fun and games. Just ask hungry, medically deprived folks in Greece, Portugal, Spain, and Cuba. It was in Cuba where I observed four-year-olds out in hot fields hand-harvesting carrots and cabbages. Many helped load transport wagons. Obviously OSHA would not approve!

Provision of required retreaters' shelters can be so simple it becomes complex. If everyone serious about these issues starts thinking and working now, there will be sufficient time to build suitable individual and family shelter and storage facilities or to develop relationships with neighbors that lead to such.

CHAPTER NINE

SECURITY

Traditionally, survivalists have assumed that sufficient anarchy would set in during an economic collapse to allow them to defend their retreats, families, and goods using uncontrolled, unaccounted-for deadly force . . . lots of unimpeded deadly force administered without any concern for answering to legal authorities. Certainly life was cheap and killing common in Somalia and Bosnia, but some of these folks are now facing international charges. Dispensing deadly force when it is not called for will definitely be a problem for 21st-century retreaters unwise enough to do so.

This helps explain why I titled this chapter "Security" rather than "Defending Your Retreat." We now have specific examples from many different countries and places pointing out that planning to shoot it out with intruders is not workable—especially in the long term, for which we must plan.

As a practical matter, this mentality never was realistic. It was mostly wishful thinking on the part of gun-owning retreaters who probably assumed such activities would be fun, interesting, and macho, as well as fair retribution against those who refused to plan or who had spent years sucking off the taxpayers through government programs they were forced to support.

I get that most retreaters are gun owners. But in order to survive we must wisely look at all issues that affect our ability to actually survive, including retreat security. And we must do this with a critical eye to actually making it through the tough times ahead.

Other than situations of absolute dictatorships and civil wars—the Soviet Union in the 1920s and '30s, where everybody was shooting everybody else on the flimsiest of pretexts; and Syria at the time of this writing, where anarchy seems to prevail—few collapsed economies have devolved to a point where society ignored the private taking of life or maiming for whatever reason. Even though street protests and riots go on frequently in present-day Greece, Spain, and Italy, penalties for using deadly force are still enforced.

Most national revolutions are political—for example, those in Cuba in the 1950s and Spain in the 1930s, both of which were very bloody. In any revolution, a sort of normalcy soon sets in, including severe to very severe retroactive penalties for previous crimes against persons and property. What we Americans face is the same as now faced by Greeks, Irish, Icelanders, Portuguese, Spanish, French, and Italians: an economic revolution/collapse. This could lead to a legal restructuring, but that is unlikely if current experience holds true.

Alan Korwin has written and published a great number of books on the subject of shooting in defense of person or property. My strong suggestion is to get your hands on these inexpensive, well-researched and -documented books and then read them carefully *before* you set up your retreat-security plan. For more information, check out his website at www.gunlaws.com.

Korwin points out that American property owners face an absolute-minimum $15,000 legal bill after an otherwise justified firearms incident—even in a self-defense situation inside your home. Should an incident be questionable, legal fees go way out of sight and reason. Not only might you have to answer to police-type authorities, but a victim's relatives may sue for wrongful death, medical costs, or endangerment. We cannot assume this legal danger will lessen during an economic collapse. It may intensify as parasites desperately search for alternate sources of funds, suing with even more abandon than they do now.

As another example, the National Rifle Association now endorses self-defense liability insurance covering up to $50,000 in legal costs to members! And some suggest that this is a floor and not a ceiling as to what a defense might run.

Firearms defense situations are especially grim out in rural America, which is exactly opposite of what you may have thought or hoped. Should your shooting incident involve nameless, faceless, urban predators, it may be accommodated out in rural America. Not overlooked or accepted but accommodated. Retreat shooters still will have unwanted legal bills, meetings with authorities, notoriety, and possible disdain from locals.

However, properly hidden, tough-to-access rural retreats will not likely be subject to predatory city people. Many urban dwellers cannot leave their cities for a great variety of reasons, including the absence of a vehicle, fuel, motivation, or specific knowledge of where exactly to go. Let's also not discount the reputation of some rural residents (somewhat self-generated) as well-armed and able and willing to shoot intruders, which might actually help keep would-be retreaters in the cities without the country folk having to fire a shot.

The chances are much better that rural retreaters may shoot a local boy or girl than an urban interloper. Then the fat is really in the fire. Local youngsters may know just enough about a reported or gossiped-about retreat to be curious about what's really going on. Lots of unfortunate circumstances can add up to a tragic ending for everyone, but especially the newcomers. The legal and perhaps medical bills will really pile up, especially if personal liability suits are filed for injury or wrongful death.

The immediate problems will be severe, but in the long run local gossip, publicity, and generally very bad feelings will destroy your retreat plans. Survivors will quickly discover that rural neighbors will ostracize them and they cannot resupply.

Defending against this youthful, adventurous curiosity is very simple. The longer you live in rural communities and the more friends and acquaintances you make, the less likely people will be overly curious about you or your retreat. Moving in with a known rural resident usually guarantees there will be no such incidents.

We once believed we could stock up and button up our retreats for six or eight months, seeing us through an emergency collapse as well as past defense requirements. Now it is evident our retreating must span four to six years, necessitating that we sometimes leave to resupply. Yet, simply disappearing until dangers pass is no longer an option. Being known and valued in the community for having a needed skill helps immensely with getting to know locals and having them trust you, leading to a relationship where you and your neighbors support and defend one another.

It has been my experience that, on average, rural residents, especially in the Midwest and South, tend to be more morally grounded than city dwellers. But exceptions are out there. Rural jealousy can be an extremely powerful force. Retreating city folks with a better-than-you attitude—who flaunt their wealth, education, past employment, good looks, expensive toys, shiny vehicles, trophy wives, or sexual proclivity—might be preyed on in one form or another by a jealous neighbor. Rural residents can be as jealous and picky as a line of chorus girls. Your actions may cause you to be shunned in a rural community, but residents generally won't resort to criminal activities or illegal acts of any kind. For example, they won't rob you.

So other issues are much more important than stockpiling firearms for defending your retreat. Guns are also, as mentioned, a very poor choice for bringing home wild game when used in sport hunting circumstances. Is there any role for guns at a retreat? Definitely.

Although retreaters may not actively hunt, some will have opportunistic chances to easily bag some wild game off the front porch or along the fence row. And guns will be necessary to keep wolves, coyotes, owls, foxes, hawks, raccoons, and other predators away from goats, chickens, ducks, or rabbits, as well as keeping them out of the cherry, apple, and peach trees. Birds in fruit orchards area also a problem, as are squirrels or raccoons tearing up attic insulation. Trapping these critters works, but shooting them is quicker and more satisfying. But exercise caution when taking action against these predators. Shooting them may be illegal and could lead to trouble for new retreaters. Be discreet. In other words, let the locals wear the hawk feathers in their hatbands, not you.

As a general rule of thumb, an arsenal consisting of a .22 rifle, shotgun, high-powered rifle, .22 pistol, and high-powered handgun would seem adequate and appropriate for most retreats. After all my admonitions about the limited value of firearms, readers might validly question why two pistols. Hopefully we have agreed that we are going to be very careful about shooting anyone even if he is caught forcibly grappling with your wife or daughter. In this traumatizing and unlikely situation, it is essential that you first ascertain whether you are dealing with a local and then fire a couple of rounds into the ceiling or air. Yet, assuming you have done everything else right, there is still a very remote possibility that the attack is real and that it threatens the safety of your family, your supplies, or even the very existence of the retreat. Shoot only when immediate consequences are much worse than future ones.

You may only have one firearm with you during an emergency, and this is often a handgun because it is portable. Smaller .22-caliber pistols are good for practice, as there is no sense wasting tough-to-replace large-bore pistol rounds on practice. Plus, retreaters are more likely to have a pistol with them when an edible target of opportunity, such as a raccoon or rabbit, comes along.

As kids growing up on the farm, we bought our .22 and shotgun ammo one round at a time at a local store. We never got used to having more than a very few rounds in our pockets. Our annual game-like contest was to see how many deer, pheasants, coons, rabbits, and quail we could collect with the fewest rounds. I recall eight deer with nine rounds per season as not uncommon.

Based on my personal use, my best estimate is that eight high-powered rifle rounds, fifty .22 rifle rounds, a half box of shotgun shells, six or eight high-powered pistol rounds, and a half box of .22 pistol rounds per year should be sufficient. This is in addition to the few rounds of ammo mentioned in the "finding value" chapter, where I discussed the limitations of planning to use ammo as trade stock.

At these rates of consumption, it is not a difficult chore to lay up enough ammo for four to six years. So many hundreds of millions of rounds of ammo along with literally tons of reloading components have been privately "laid back" that I personally believe there will never be a true shortage of ammo in this country. Though at present wild surges in demand for ammo have caused some large dealers, including Walmart, to limit purchases.

This flies in the face of genuine, well-meaning but inexperienced retreaters who really want to believe they are going to have to run their retreats like some sort of Israeli military outpost. My question is, who are you going to shoot it out with? Even in a totally collapsed economy, government agents who identify someone as a target can always bring much more force to bear than retreaters can ever muster. This is especially true in 21st-century situations, where retreaters may be demonized into popular adversaries by bureaucrats out to prove their superiority and the necessity of their bringing you to justice and enhancing their budgets. Think of Ruby Ridge and Waco in this regard.

Many survivors currently assume that they will run their operations like military camps. This is not a workable or reliable assumption. What retreat family or group, I often ask, will accept casualties as a result of military-like actions? Especially among our sons and daughters? Securing an area involves sending out patrols to make certain all is secure. Whom in your group are you going to send out?

So what is truly effective for retreat security? Note the use of "security," which is proactive, rather than "defense," which is, of course, after the fact, defensive. This signifies a major new 21st-century paradigm for many of us.

As preached in virtually every chapter so far, proper security has to involve three things—obscurity, obscurity, obscurity! In that exact order. Of course, in keeping with the redundancy rule exhorted throughout this book, how you orchestrate this obscurity could easily have three or six or eight different components.

As an absolute fallback—true in many more cases than we might initially suspect—many survivors are planning to use parts

B, C, or even D of their shelter program as part of their security obscurity. In other words, a van or travel camper may be stacked with supplies and parked far away in an alternate, secure location to be reached in an emergency. Placing a number of secure emergency caches in your area may also be necessary. It may be costly, but the best security may be that you and your family are not home when danger arrives.

All this implies that successful retreats be reasonably difficult to get to and low profile—definitely not shining examples of "here's lots of free stuff—come and get it!" Being way out of town—at least five miles—so that potential plunderers either cannot sneak up on foot or must drive up in an easily recognized vehicle helps immeasurably.

Several retreaters in more densely populated areas of the eastern U.S. plan large, appropriately colored signs warning of severe nuclear radiation danger at their sites. They also plan to display official-looking letters claiming government agents have impounded and closed the area because of both radiation and asbestos contamination. It is essential in this situation to keep signs of life—including coming and going—at the retreat to a minimum. Some rural retreaters also post pistol targets on their front door or window out in plain sight. Perhaps you don't want to shoot someone, but you do want potentially dangerous intruders to believe that you could.

Locking the gate to your retreat fence only works when the retreat cannot be seen from the gate. Otherwise visitors, especially friendly ones, will just hop over fences and gates to walk to the retreat. And don't forget, in our 21st-century reality, we cannot button up for the duration!

At this writing, cutting taxes, reducing spending, raising taxes, and other such measures won't work to head off economic catastrophes we see ahead. Greece has raised taxes, and it isn't working. Spain and Portugal are reducing spending dramatically, and that isn't working. France is increasing taxes and spending, and we won't have to wait long to see how that is working out for them.

Only massively cutting rules and regulations similar to what Germany did five or six years ago will work to restore our economy. International examples are especially good in this regard. Think of the Baltic nations of Latvia, Lithuania, and Estonia, as well as Great Britain under Margaret Thatcher.

Like most survivors, I earnestly hope and pray our society's many incentive-reducing, work-impeding, mollycoddling, dependence-producing, and wealth-destroying rules and regulations will disappear during a crash. That would make living four or six years as retreaters almost worthwhile. Yet, based on what we see in Italy, Portugal, Spain, France, Greece, Ireland, Iceland, and other nations yet to be identified, the best we can presently hope for is that many of the most onerous rules and regulations will *not* be enforced. This may simply occur because enforcing bureaucrats have not been paid and cannot be paid. They simply don't come to work and are thus unavailable to enforce rules and regulations. This is exactly what's happening right now in Greece and Spain. But, as mentioned, never assume that these onerous, unnecessary, petty rules and regulations will not be used against retreaters, and often in an arbitrary manner. It is best to keep violations a very deep, dark secret.

Hungry, lazy bureaucrats may demand bribes, which with no other source of income, is a logical result. Think of Mexican police in this regard. But if retreaters start on this slippery slope, greedy bureaucrats will soon break them.

Our best security hope is obscurity combined with community friendship and support. In some instances, allowing thieves to abscond with some supplies may be cheaper and smarter than resisting. These are more areas of intense contemplation for new retreaters to research and consider.

CHAPTER TEN

MEDICAL

The earth beneath our traditional preparedness medical plans has shifted dramatically within the last six or eight years. In some ways, the shift is even more significant than other changes with which 21st-century retreaters must contend. As a result, planning a completely effective rule of threes survival medical program may no longer be possible or practical. This was always a difficult area for most retreaters. Now, at best, it will be extremely difficult—even for those who start early with ample funds.

There is hope, as a few work-around strategies are still out there. Mastering these will be especially important, given new 21st-century circumstances that will drive many of our retreating survival plans. For instance, the population in the United States is aging. Aging retreaters require a great deal more medical services and medications than younger ones. This is certainly not a profound observation, but it is one that many have not considered in their preparedness plans.

Consider also that, in a huge number of cases, aging retreaters—already financially secure—often move into rural areas, where they establish retreats. Often these older folks intend that their children and grandchildren will join them after life in the cities or suburbs becomes intolerable. These older folks may feel they are moving back to their roots, or they may simply seek a less-intense rural atmosphere. Establishing retreats may currently be secondary in these folks' thinking, but this could change very quickly.

This in part drives the need to solve medical services and supply issues, especially for young city families moving in with aged parents or relatives. This is a difficult obligation wherein we attempt to make life as comfortable as possible for older people who are making life possible for the next generation or two by providing rural retreat opportunities.

Prior to our new 21st-century medical reality, the rule of threes for survivors often relied on foreign meds that may have included mail order delivery, veterinary supplies, and what may be termed "conventional supplies," from local druggists in one form or pretext or another using duplicate prescription forms.

This approach has been made more difficult in the last few years by the worldwide war on illicit drugs, which has made securing medical supplies outside governmentally sanctioned systems increasingly harder. It is no longer possible, for instance, to just walk in and purchase many prescription medications over the counter in Mexico, Puerto Rico, and other places. We also see from experiences in other countries that government-sanctioned supplies of medicines quickly evaporate under extreme national financial stress.

However, some solutions are still available. Don't give up. Read on and be prepared to use creativity and energy when solving this problem. One quick example is 222s, a mild yet very effective painkiller containing 8 mg of codeine, which is still available over the counter in Canada at very reasonable prices. Although Mexico and Puerto Rico have tightened pharmaceutical rules and regulations, it is still possible to purchase most nonnarcotic meds there without prescriptions. Two cultural realities help. First, most pharmacies in these places will generally accept what we might term somewhat borderline homemade prescriptions. Second, Mexican and Puerto Rican druggists—anxious to make profits on sales—will often accept a gratuity in exchange for a nice large order of meds, paid in cash. It takes a bit of finessing, including becoming friends with *farmacia* employees, but it is being done as we speak—especially away from border cities in little sleepy rural burgs. That we can no longer order meds by mail from pharmacies in Greece, Mexico, England, the Philippines, and even Thailand is a real issue for survivors.

Ecuador and Thailand are about the only two reliable places remaining where just about any medicines can be purchased over the counter without a prescription, both far too distant for most American retreaters to take advantage of. And bringing realistic long-term supplies back through U.S. Customs is not easy. Generally in person or by mail, U.S. Customs permits three-month supplies of medicines across our border. Above that amount, officials consider them to be "not for personal use."

Greece and Spain, once excellent places to look for mail order and over-the-counter supplies, are especially grim examples today. This is a direct result of government programs and economic collapse. Very few to no meds are manufactured in Greece or Spain today. Most were imported through government-sponsored medical programs. After a year or more of not paying for these imported supplies, many exporting nations and drug companies simply turned off the tap. Currently, the few medications that are available are smuggled into these countries or provided by charitable organizations. Of course, the cost for the few available drugs is ruinously high.

The situation in Cuba became so bad that young children literally begged for vitamins and other medicines that tourists had with them. Rather than working to replace Castro and his henchmen, brain-dead Canadian tourists thought it their duty to haul vast troves of vitamins, among many other goods, in their luggage to Cuba for distribution to the "poor unfortunates" while blaming America for the sorry condition of the Cuban rank and file.

Even in places where vital medicines are manufactured in country, they may not be available for purchase. Medical systems in all collapsed economies are under strict government control—a direction in which our country is rapidly heading.

Without government funds to purchase from manufacturers, national drug companies either quit making drugs or produce only for export. In many instances, governments simply confiscate drug company products, which quickly leads to no meds at all. Currently, that is the situation in Venezuela. Same old same old: all medications are free, but there aren't any, unless one is part of the ruling elite. This argues mightily for stockpiling now while medicines are still available.

Of course, when stockpiling anything, you have to consider shelf life of the item. This is a little tricky with drugs. Several years ago a study (the Shelf Life Extension Program, or SLEP) by the Federal Food and Drug Administration for the U.S. Department of Defense established that virtually all non-narcotic meds retain their effectiveness for at least 20 years. The results of this study were published in several papers and periodicals, including the *Wall Street Journal*, which is where I read it. Conventional wisdom (plus expiration dates on the containers of filled medicines) has always suggested that we should use prescription drugs in a year or less. But according to this federal study, this caution had no basis in reality. SLEP found that some drugs stay fresh for years longer than their expiration dates, thus enabling the military to save millions of dollars in replacing expired drugs.

This brings us to an absolute iron rule of survival meds: never attempt to secure any narcotic-type drugs or painkillers using homemade prescriptions or bribes in established pharmacies. Absolutely no sales of narcotics will ever be made without checking into the validity of the prescriptions. Such scrutiny often includes phone calls to the doctor's office listed on prescriptions at the buyer's expense, even from Mexico. Additionally, be well aware that all narcotic-type meds have very short shelf lives. Storing for any length of time will not work. Unlike other drugs, narcotics just die, right there on the shelf—often in two years or less.

Using modern computers and scanners to produce good, credible, workable prescriptions is not rocket science. That's why, before filling any narcotic prescription, druggists first call the doctor's office about that specific prescription. It also explains why so many modern prescriptions are done by fax or phone rather than paper carried in person to a pharmacy.

Using reproduction prescriptions in small rural community pharmacies is generally not a problem so long as you're not seeking narcotics, the prescriptions are of good quality, and quantities requested are reasonable—usually no more than a three-month supply. Everyone knows everyone else in small, tight-knit rural enclaves. As a result, drugs are dispensed on the basis of knowing individuals as well as the paper itself.

You may even be able to use duplicates up and down the street. This is especially possible when dealing with pharmacies in grocery supermarkets, super stores, and nameless, faceless big-box outlets. These must be cash purchases that do not appear on insurance claims, private or government. For instance, a local techie with aging, somewhat infirm parents who require frequent meds makes it a practice to never use an original prescription. Using numerous exact copies has become a game for him. Caution however—some recent prescription forms display as invalid even when scanned rather than photocopied. It is better to test first. Everything changes, especially technology!

Currently both copy-protected and older standard prescription forms are out there. Other than in places like Mexico and Argentina, where they don't care, we soon won't be able to copy prescription forms for personal use. Absolutely no prescription should ever pass through your hands without being scanned and saved in a personal computer—another rule of practical survival meds. Copying may not be possible, but duplicating by using a scanner may still be an option.

That leaves veterinary supplies. Access to veterinarian supplies of meds has been tightened up dramatically in recent years, perhaps because of survivalists' interest in them. Some good, basic materials—mostly valuable for treating wounds and infections, as well as trauma situations—are still available. But most complex medicines, when used in a veterinarian context, are now heavily restricted. Also animals don't usually require increasingly complex meds, which are now more and more common in humans. However, let's not forget that farm and vet supplies are a wonderful source of inexpensive disinfectants, wound dressings, fungus and skin treatments, bug sprays, and such unrestricted supplies.

But essentially another leg of our traditional rule of threes medicine preparations is gone. As mentioned, government takeover of purchase and distribution of drugs, including veterinary medical supplies, is much more onerous than virtually anything else on the medical front. This is off the scope of most people but still a very real problem, as illustrated by what's happening in Cuba, Ireland, Greece, Spain, and Italy. When governments go broke and can no longer pay their bills, vital medical supplies wither and die, and often very quickly, catching many folks completely by surprise.

Can't happen in the United States, you say? It couldn't happen in prosperous modern Europe either, could it?

As rural retreaters get to know their local medical providers, both licensed official and skilled unofficial, they can put together a future medical storage program. Such a program could run as follows.

Mention to those you know in local medical professions that quantity discounts may be available for the purchase of needed meds and that you wish to purchase while funds are available. In my experience, the necessary paper is always forthcoming. Assembling sufficient quantities may entail taking duplicate prescriptions up and down the street. If so, so be it. Be reasonable about quantities requested at any one pharmacy and never try this with painkillers.

Frequently, rural retreaters can trade with medical people: your carpentry, fiberglassing, welding, or small-engine repair skills for their prescriptions or the medicines themselves. Extra garden produce also makes good trading stock. But this only works after long periods of intense, in-depth acclimation to an area. If you relocated to the area because of close family or friends, they may have already established this relationship with the medical community.

Dentistry has always been a big issue for retreaters, and nothing much has changed in that area. Because only minimal amounts of dental supplies are usually required, some dental work will be available in rural areas during a collapse. Here skill trumps supply, allowing some work to be done. Emergency dental work may involve travel and some relatively high fees, but it will probably be available.

Most folks who have become retreaters, either by choice or under duress without prior planning, report that the best dental plan is proactive work undertaken well before a collapse. Of course, this won't accommodate accidents and injuries, such as breaking a tooth on a piece of shot, but it does prevent many routine dental emergencies. Talk to your dentist now, particularly if you have dental insurance, about things you can legitimately do now to reduce your dental needs in the future. One thing that comes to mind is to replace large amalgam fillings with acrylic fillings, which are less inclined to swell and split a tooth later on.

We can hope, but not necessarily assume, that a healthier lifestyle out in the sticks may do away with or lower doses of blood pressure, upset stomach, and cholesterol medications, to name just a few quick examples, thus stretching supplies. That certainly will be a factor as we watch less TV, get more exercise, and lose weight on the bland to very bland foods we'll have to eat.

There is also some hope that, as our government medical system goes bust, more and more common generic medications will be offered over the counter without doctor's orders. This may not be a generous act on the part of our benevolent bureaucracy as much as a way to extend dwindling funds used to pay for medications. This is a result of the general rule that over-the-counter medicines and preparations are not covered by Medicare, other government programs, or even by some insurance plans. In other words, purchase of many currently restricted meds on the part of citizens may be made possible to conserve government funds because these meds will be cleared for over-the-counter sales.

We can only hope that a worrisome lump will not show up during the four to six years of our retreat. If one does, we can only hope local medical people will be up to the task of dealing with it. We should never assume that there will be no medical specialists among rural retreaters. Doctors, physician assistants, dentists, and nurses are also retreaters.

It might be helpful here to remind you to lay in a supply of ordinary but necessary medical or health items peculiar to your circumstances: extra prescription eye glasses, personal medical maintenance items from insulin to catheters to an extra hernia truss to a supply of contact lenses—whatever you use on a regular basis. And in this vein, note that a lot of health aid items are available disposable or reusable, and a mix of both might be practical (e.g., needles, catheters, contact lenses, over-the-counter meds, etc.).

As mentioned going in, planning for adequate medical services and medicines is really tough for 21st-century retreaters. There are no easy, one-size-fits-all answers out there. Medical care will not be much of an issue for retreaters who are fortunate enough to enjoy good health (or don't suffer any injuries) or those who have done extensive preplanning for their medical needs. Lots more scheming, planning, and preparation are needed in this area for most of us.

CHAPTER ELEVEN

EQUIPMENT AND SUPPLIES

Finally we arrive at a segment of 21st-century retreating that hasn't changed all that much. There are some changes to be sure, mostly brought on by advances in technology, plus the need for longer-term planning. But many preppers will find this chapter to be at least somewhat familiar.

Advances in technology have brought those of us who live in the country easier lives and, most significantly, equipment and supplies that have longer shelf lives and do not require nearly as much care and maintenance. On the down side, lots of our survival equipment has shifted from requiring semiskilled to skilled maintenance.

I think of my old, long-departed Russian grandmother, *babushka*. We once asked her which of her modern kitchen appliances was her favorite. This was just after the introduction of microwave ovens, electric coffee grinders, single-line phone service, vacuum cleaners, and other appliances that cost less than $800 each. It took this lady, who had grown old using wood-fired kitchen ranges, only a nanosecond to identify indoor running water as her favorite kitchen "appliance." And, as a quick afterthought, *hot and cold indoor running water.*

Of course, it's all in one's perspective, which speaks volumes about past experiences and circumstances, perhaps identifying why we each are as we are.

The information and opinions that follow may not be entirely relevant to survival. They may not always apply to the rule of threes, unless readers wish to make that application. All definitely do apply to eventually making it in rural America, mostly based on my 70-plus years of living in rural to extremely rural areas of the United States and other places around the globe. At a time, for relatively short intervals, I also lived in several medium to very large cities, many where English was not the preferred language.

Having seen many city people up close and personal trying to make it in the country, I have observed some tragically foolish situations, where the foolishness was obvious and preventable had these good folks either been willing to listen or abandon a stubborn course of action that was eating them alive. Bottom line, with a foot in both types of societies, I believe I am in a valid position to comment on how to integrate into rural communities. Other than to mention that folks new to rural life might nab a copy of my book *Starting a New Life in Rural America*, available from Paladin Press, I will press on to general information and issues pertaining to tools, equipment, and supplies that new rural retreaters need to consider.

More than just "the devil is in the details," all this has much to do with each and every retreater's personal circumstance. No two of us are ever alike. General issues of equipment and supplies necessary to implement your rule-of-threes program quickly sort themselves out into exactly what tools and supplies will be essential for each category of vital need. In other words, what equipment is needed to heat your retreat; store and use water; process and store food; produce some light (allowing vital work to go on after short winter days); transport, store, and use emergency supplies; keep critters at bay; trade service and skills with neighbors; and perform thousands of other similar tasks mostly related to maintaining your rule of threes.

First let's look at the really large issue of equipment that applies to all categories of survival needs simultaneously. I expect this will generate some heated reactions.

A basic concept of country living involves the unavoidable conclusion that unless newcomers are very careful to mechanize their retreats, they will quickly become forced-labor camps. You will never catch up with vital chores that absolutely needed to be done yesterday. This precept immediately precedes one that informs us that, if you don't have anything immediately pressing to do around the retreat, you just don't understand the situation.

New retreaters absolutely must mechanize as quickly as possible. This is costly, often with long, arduous learning curves, but it must be done. As a quick example, every time our neighbor comes over with his tractor to borrow a tractor-mounted tool, we must first spend half an hour tightening bolts, adjusting brakes and clutch, replacing bulbs, and doing other maintenance on his machine. He is getting better at maintaining his machine, but slowly, slowly.

Spading a large garden plot by hand, for instance, is a nonstarter. So is hand-mowing around your retreat, which is necessary to keep critters away and abate fire danger. Splitting sufficient firewood is best done with mechanical assistance. Think also of generating enough electricity to keep refrigerators, freezers, and well pumps operational. Perhaps it will be necessary to plow snow; move heavy equipment, supplies, and fuel drums; or lift machinery for repair, logs, or moving. Mechanization will make these chores much easier and efficient.

TRACTOR

Purchasing separate pieces of motorized equipment—such as power mowers, wood splitters, and rototillers—to accomplish all these hundreds of tasks seems simpler and initially less expensive. But it is *never* wise. Maintenance problems become severe, spare part inventories become a nightmare, and most important, these little individual mowers, tillers, generators, and even log splitters are cheaply built homeowner models. They will not withstand four to six years of earnest use. The total cost when it's all said and done will exceed the cost to purchase a small tractor and attachable tools.

Your best option is a smaller 20- to 30-horsepower diesel tractor onto which dozens of special-purpose tools can be quickly and easily mounted. As a bonus, special-purpose, laborsaving, tractor-mounted tools can often be purchased in rural areas in very good used condition. And they need not all be bought the same year a retreat is opened. Most specialized tractor tools are accommodated on common three-point tractor mounts. You simply back up and insert three pins and a power take-off shaft—not that this doesn't take some practice, but eventually you learn the procedure.

Kubota, John Deere, and New Holland all make serviceable four-wheel-drive diesel models. Choose diesel rather than gas because diesel tractors are more powerful and require far less maintenance. They run forever if supplied with easy-to-handle red diesel and proper engine oil, filters, and lube. Four-wheel-drive is necessary to take full advantage of *all* your tractor's power. You probably should consider only tractors with hydraulic bucket loaders, which are essential to move heavy loads about the retreat.

As previously mentioned, tax-exempt red diesel fuel usually sells for a bit less than gasoline. Diesel, not gas, might be available from a local farmer on a resupply basis. Gallon for gallon, diesel is far more powerful than gasoline. In fact, many farmers no longer store gasoline on their farms at all.

Freestanding diesel generators are out there, but they are uncommon. Mounting a diesel generator to a tractor is easy. More power is generated from larger tractor engines, and fuel consumption is usually substantially less than with self-contained, freestanding generator units.

Because of longer time spans for which we must plan to retreat, we will have to leave from time to time to try to scrounge up fuel, food, parts, and supplies. This could be as ordinary and simple as a vital three-quarter-inch bolt and nut. Ideally, leaving would be done in a small to medium diesel-powered truck. Unfortunately, no small diesel trucks are currently available in the United States, though some very nice Toyota and Isuzu diesel trucks are available in Mexico and Canada. Importation is possible but not quick, easy, or cheap. We do have the promise of a medium-sized diesel truck from Chrysler, but at this writing, nothing is forthcoming. All we can do is hope that something shows up soon. Very soon!

Three-quarter-ton diesel trucks are out there, but they suffer mightily from the "toos"—too expensive to purchase, too expensive to operate, and too large to maneuver easily for most retreat chores. Older small diesel trucks in acceptable condition may still be available. We used a diesel Isuzu at our rural retreat for many years. When it was finally old and decrepit, we traded it, not realizing it was irreplaceable.

A few diesel cars are now available in this country. Some might be pressed into service, pulling trailers or used as tote wagons. Watch out for new small diesel cars that are built like fine watches and have pesky little things that break, or that are not built sturdily enough to withstand the rigors of unpaved roads on a daily basis.

A diesel tractor pulling a small trailer might handle your hauling chores at the retreat. This arrangement is good for firewood, drums of diesel fuel, sacks of corn, and other things. Small tractors get up to 15 mph on the highway. Back on the farm, as a kid, that's how we (and other farming families) went to town. We are much richer today. Even in agricultural communities, you seldom see tractors on the road or in town hauling families.

GENERATOR

A generator is next in the line of larger multiple-use tools required at a retreat. Tractor-driven generators are, as mentioned, the hands-down best option for retreat electricity.

Right now many people in Greece and Spain are having their electric power and phone service cut off for nonpayment. Life without a phone at a retreat is doable, but not without some source of electricity. In a prolonged crisis, will our electric power be cut off or, more likely, spike up in price so much we can't afford it? We can't know for sure, so it is best to plan for the worst.

Quick, inexpensive, easy methods of evaluating your generator capacity needs, hook-up procedures, servicing requirements, likely spare parts, service tools, etc., have been covered in many other books. Again, there is no need to replow that ground, other than to strongly suggest preparedness folks need a generator large enough to power water pumps, freezers, some small tools, and lights, though not necessarily all running at the same time.

Note that we definitely do not intend to cook or heat water with electricity generated at our retreat. Plans for these chores must include a source other than home-produced electricity, which, even when done with diesel tractors, is fantastically inefficient and costly.

How about propane—useful but not absolutely essential for food preparation and processing garden produce? Retreaters in rural Mexico, Argentina, and Iceland had continuing access to propane. Many retreaters stock a two- to three-year supply in a 1,000-gallon tank. They may also use this supply to fill 5-gallon tanks. Will retreaters in rural areas of this country be able to re-supply propane? Given the surplus of natural gas now produced, there probably will be some sources of supply. Propane is not the same as liquefied natural gas, but one may push the other into wider availability. We don't know.

CHAIN SAW

Another expensive, often difficult-to-master piece of equipment that perhaps 90 percent of rural retreats must have is the chain saw. It is possible to cut enough wood by hand with which to cook and heat—after all, people have done it for generations and are still doing it in some places—but it is an onerous task for the long haul, especially for people who aren't used to hard, physical labor. There is a lot of good information out there in books and online sites about chain saws as well. Let's leave this as another research project for you to complete, other than mentioning that you should collect extra files, chains, air filters, starter ropes, and other parts before the hour of serious need arrives. In my opinion, only Stihl and Husqvarna make saws sufficiently long-lived and rugged for retreaters.

HAND TOOLS

It is hoped that new retreaters will have sufficient time to establish exactly which pliers, socket sets, wrenches, screw drivers, hammers, vise grips, punches, cold chisels, and other tools will be needed. Those using propane should figure out exactly which hand tools they require. Some are specialized, requiring lots of prior experience to use and maintain efficiently.

This list may seem foolishly slim to you. But even a very comprehensive list will miss many tools that, depending on your circumstances, could be vital. Only four or five years of experience will demonstrate which tools will be essential to you. Also in many cases, you can borrow needed tools from neighbors, provided that you have taken the time to develop cordial relations with them and that you return them promptly and in good condition. I lend tools frequently.

MISCELLANEOUS AND SPARE PARTS

Additionally, there are grease cartridges, grease guns, oil and oil spouts, oil filters, fuses, tire stems, tire gauges, air cleaners and filters, fuel filters, hydraulic filters, and other items that are required to keep retreat equipment operational. You might also include some replacement wear parts for tractor tools such as mowers, plows, and pumps.

Tires for the tractor and truck can be an issue. Be sure they are all fairly new as you head into a potential collapse. Trailer and tractor tires last 20-plus years unless damaged by inexperienced users.

Barrel taps, bungs, spanner wrenches, haul chains, clean empty barrels, large tanks, pumps, nozzles, hoses, and other items will be needed to access and deploy fuel.

Some repair and old-fashioned production equipment may be difficult to find in today's high-tech society. As an example, when was the last time you shopped for ax, maul, or shovel replacement handles, maul handle cleats, steel splitting wedges, falling wedges, and tools? Last winter I spent days looking for a high-quality steel felling wedge to replace one I had lost on the job! Most farm supply stores and some hardware stores in rural areas will carry these items. Stock up on them now since they may fall subject to shortages and be hard to find when you need them most desperately.

CUTTING TOOLS

In my experience, first-time rural retreaters frequently overlook cutting tools. In addition to a variety of good knives, think tin snips, hack saws, extra Sawzall blades, axes, files and sharpening stones to sharpen blades, and for other uses. These are all items I frequently lend to neighbors.

PERSONAL ITEMS

Rough, physical, outdoor work requires boots, gloves, rain gear, hats, jackets, rugged pants, tough work shoes, and more. Stock up on these while they are still available.

HOUSEHOLD ITEMS

Processing food, either for freezers or canning, requires large pots, plastic bags, freezer tape, propane stoves, tubs, jars, lids, magic markers, and whatever else you might usefully collect before a collapse. Caring for the garden will require hoses, hose repair parts, couplings, nozzles, sprinklers, fertilizer, pesticides, and seeds, as well as experience in how to use these items.

I have touched only lightly on a great many extremely important issues here. The only way to know for sure what all is needed is to spend time at your retreat being self-sufficient. In that regard, a neighbor (I have no close neighbors) sometimes stops by to borrow a large pipe wrench or other special tool he does not have. That's OK—he hasn't been at this long enough to know what all he needs, and all tools are quickly returned in perfect condition. He adds to his tool inventory as his budget allows, and someday I might have to ask him for a favor.

Only by relocating to a rural retreat early on will the average inexperienced city person be able to figure out what he doesn't know and take steps to correct his own situation. I find that listing broad categories of equipment and tool needs is helpful, whereas being too specific is problematic. Something important will likely be overlooked, often something *very* important. I think of a forgotten pocket calculator desperately needed out on a project on the far, cold, barren Aleutians Islands. We would have been home a miserable day sooner if we had not forgotten a simple little three-dollar pocket calculator. We didn't need the pocket calculator ourselves. It was younger guys who had been to government school and couldn't do long division by hand who needed one.

Lots of good how-to information is out there for you to find and study. Experience is always a good, albeit sometimes rough, teacher. Novice retreaters must figure out what they don't know and what they need to acquire before the situation gets really serious. Then they must research, research, research!

CHAPTER TWELVE

EMPLOYMENT AND RETIREMENT RELATIVE TO THE RULE OF THREES

Individual readers will have to decide whether the following information and observations apply only to survival or more broadly to their lives in general. Perhaps they apply to neither, but that's a personal call. As in the past, survival in the 21st century remains an intensely personal matter.

Much of this started as personal observations of friends and acquaintances who found that after retiring they couldn't make it financially. We have already noted that it is amazing how little we can live on when circumstances dictate. Yet many of these folks were unable or unwilling to adapt their lifestyles to their new economic reality and found themselves in tragically hopeless situations.

Personal responsibility still applies, but no matter whether it's survival/retreating or just retiring, this personal responsibility flows back significantly more years than people suspect. In other words, those who put off vital decisions of planning, educating themselves, saving, and investing till the end of their careers will find they must labor much more intently than those who started this process decades before. This "retirement process" involves more than just investing in a pension or retirement savings plan; it also applies to employment, education, and lifestyle choices.

Personally, I have no plans to ever retire. Nevertheless, plans and procedures can demonstrably make life easier and more comfortable. We can also easily see that observing an employment rule of threes in a rural survival/retreat context is vital . . . not merely important, but vital.

I will start with retirement related to the rule of threes.

Restating the issue more specifically: if a certain level of income is necessary to maintain life and happiness during your later years, you had better plan at least three separate and distinct methods of providing that income. Also, believe it or not, at least one of those plans should be renewable! Renewable finances, as in growing a financial garden? Not exactly. Dividends from stock investments or interest from savings are two quick examples of renewable finances that come to mind. But can you count on these in a SHTF scenario? Certainly not. There are other income sources that are more reliable in a collapsed or depressed economy, such as providing skilled labor, trading survival goods at a profit, and hiring out your tractor and driver, tools, and whatever else you can think of.

People who think about this issue generally plan to live out their lives on funds from pensions, Social Security, or savings accounts; the sale of some accumulated assets; savings from downsizing or moving in with the kids; or perhaps earnings from skilled labor—the kind that comes with old age. Public pensions and Social Security are government programs, and we all know where our government is headed financially. We already can see the bitter end of our Social Security system. And if not the end, at least dramatically reduced payments are to be expected. We also know that government pensions—municipal, state, and national—are dramatically overpromised and underfunded. As our society becomes more broke, there simply will not be funds available to pay out at promised levels. While we have seen this to be true in Greece, Spain, and Portugal, it is also currently the situation in Illinois, California, and Michigan.

Many private pension plans are also seriously overextended and underfunded in the United States. During the past few years, many employers have moved away from defined-benefit plans (also referred to as fully loaded plans, where you work so many years and then receive guaranteed income and other benefits determined by years of service, age at retirement, and salary). Instead, more and more companies are opting for defined- contribution plans, such as the 401(k) for new salaried employees, which puts the responsibility of investing in the hands of the employee. This requires great personal responsibility on the part of the employees to make sure their funds are wisely and effectively used. (Many states are also switching from defined-benefit to defined-contribution pension plans.) Some companies opt not to participate in any retirement plans for their employees. Among these, a few offer lump-sum cash payment to retirees, which they must then steward on their own. (As an aside, neither my father nor either of my grandfathers retired with pensions or lump-sum awards.)

The bad news is that folks relying on Social Security and pension income during their latter days will have to find other sources of income. The good news is that, until our country in general drops back well below 50 percent of its citizens living on government largesse, we won't turn our situation around. Frédéric Bastiat, a French economist and philosopher, who championed private property, free trade, and limited government, first promulgated this philosophy in the 1850s. Bastiat's teachings against governmental plundering that reallocates resources and often has ruinous unintended consequences in the long term have more recently been substantiated in numerous studies by world-class economists, as well as by economic history.

When our government goes broke and there is no money to pay promised Social Security and pensions benefits, it will get extremely ugly, especially in our nation's cities. And it will probably happen surprisingly fast. That is exactly what we currently see in many European Union nations. So what is to be done? On a personal level, retreaters must reestablish the ethic of personal responsibility by implementing a rule-of-three financial program.

More generally and collectively, we can ask that all of us work longer into our last years. Improved health and longevity make this possible. Recall that when Social Security was first implemented in 1935, the average life expectancy from birth was about 58 years for men and 62 for women. With the minimum age for receiving full retirement benefits set at age 65, the government expected most of us to pay in during our lifetimes but die before collecting. In this regard, can we really reset retirement ages up to 74 and beyond? Not in this current political atmosphere wherein many average Americans want to live at the expense of others.

Without a national policy, individually electing to work longer into our last years won't help the country as a whole. But doing so, especially when government programs go in the tank, will materially help those individuals who extended their work years. Working longer and investing wisely what little may remain of government and private pensions and lump-sum cash programs will dramatically help. But, as a result, all of us survivors will have to pick successful investments, which may include everything from buying rental properties to working gravel pits to placing our funds with experts in successful growth funds.

Using fund managers costs investors a percent or two that could be theirs if they learned to invest on their own. But this is not an easy task for anyone in a free-falling economy. In what, for instance, are you going to invest in Spain, Greece, or Portugal that makes any sense? The answer may be in German stocks and bonds or British and U.S. multinational companies. But you have to choose those shrewdly. It might be wiser to pay a professional who monitors the markets closely.

An extremely successful female investor acquaintance points out that successfully investing half a million dollars is a one-day-a-week job. Two million takes four hours each and every day, just to stay ahead of everything. For six million, it's a full-time job, plus one employee.

Another golden rule of investing: individuals must, at a minimum, invest in six stocks, six bonds, or six pieces of real estate. Obviously investing in six gravel pits or six plumbing shops is not practical. Yet, in general, you must spread risks, not knowing ahead which are dogs and which are winners. Run with the winners and ruthlessly cull the losers. Usually this entails more than a few thousand dollars of investment. Again, this argues for an early start on your investments.

So, our retiree has some Social Security, a government or

perhaps private pension, plus some investment cash on which to rely for income. This is not enough, but keep in mind that many Americans don't have even that much. Then there are any possible savings you may have, withdrawing small amounts only as absolutely needed. No sense expounding on this one, as numerous experts have already done so.

I know of a man who two different times inherited three million dollars. Each time it took him between one and two years to blow through the entire three million—one would have thought by the second three mil he would have learned, but no such luck. Probably all of us have known of or heard of such an individual or circumstance.

As a last option for retirement funds, we have some sort of self-developed employment gimmick or hustle, as many folks call it, that can lead to a bit of additional income during our later years. Perhaps this is not enough to live on but is enough when combined with other income. Ideally you should strive to make each separate component of your income rule of threes provide enough income to live on if need be.

This hustle can vary all over the landscape, including selling produce at a farmer's market booth or stand, raising and selling Christmas trees or trees for saw logs, selling salvaged building products, consulting, repairing clocks or watches, gunsmithing, making cabinets or furniture, repairing small engines, welding, snow plowing, hauling trash, and whatever else your fertile imagination can bring up. Most of these small businesses take years to develop, but once firmly in place, they can be surprisingly lucrative and steady.

This brings us right up to issues of employment in general and rural survival/retreat employment specifically. Among the Amish folks around whom I was raised, it was an item of faith that anyone past age 14 had at least two distinct employment situations based in the home. And when someone in town employed them for wages, they tried to maintain a total of three separate employment incomes, two at home and one in town.

Wives, unmarried girls, and older widows also kept at least

two different sources of employment. Usually these women zeroed in on window washing, house cleaning or sitting, pet care, butchering and processing of small poultry or small livestock, baby sitting, sewing and tailoring, leather working, interior painting and decorating, and/or bookkeeping, as well as some catering done in cooperation with other women. This, of course, is only a partial list of services these women offered in their communities. (As an aside, our daughter made excellent, almost unreasonable, money cleaning houses at a time of great financial stress in her life. Later on, at the urging of her husband, she retired from that business.)

Raising organic produce has been a veritable boon for many of these Amish women. To some skeptics, organic produce has no demonstrable superiority over regular produce, except psychological. Some see it as a gigantic scam wherein they can sell shriveled, buggy, inferior produce at inflated prices. Others swear by its health and environmental benefits. As times get tough, survivors have to be aware that this industry will likely suffer and might disappear in some areas.

Amish men undertook contract or hourly truck, tractor, and car mechanics; plumbing; electrical work; welding; construction jobs; masonry; and contract agricultural services, such as spraying, mowing, and hay baling. Others made good money taking care of farm chores while the owners or regular workers vacationed or were unavailable for work. Still others brokered fancy hardwoods, hay, tobacco, cotton, animal skins, horses, or other such products or services. Again, this list is far from complete of the opportunities out there to make supplemental money.

Teens, girls and boys, contracted to put up hay, clean barns or other outbuildings, paint barns and sheds, cut and sell firewood, remove trees, raise calves, and build fences, along with dozens of other chores and tasks. These folks always had a minimum of two distinct ways of generating income, and these services were usually done for cash only.

Retreaters new to rural economies will call it "operating in the underground economy." Soon they come to understand how widespread and common this economy really is. Excellent books on the subject of operating in the underground economy are out there, including two from Paladin (my own *Ragnar's Guide to the Underground Economy* and *Deep Inside the Underground Economy*).

Another often-unseen bonus came up when retirement age arrived, and it was time then to pick the easiest and most profitable retirement jobs. After 50 years of doing odd and second jobs off the books, it was very obvious which ones were profitable and which ones they did very well. By that time, the choice was obvious because they had already established their clientele in a couple of different businesses.

For multiple reasons already covered, new rural retreaters will have to pick up on two or three hustles." Their financial and social positions will depend on it, both now and in later years. As a result, we arrive back at the understanding that workers are most successful when they create an in-demand product or service. Then, when retirement arrives, your three alternate means of income—most of which were not even touched on in these few pages—will be in place.

Does this sound suspiciously like people living on a desert island who take in each other's washing and ironing? This is only workable in any closed economy if you believe in perpetual motion. No new wealth is created.

Rural agricultural areas produce tremendous amounts of new wealth annually from the ground up, and some production will continue after a collapse. We know this from real-life experiences in Greece, Portugal, and Cuba. Unlike our isolated island example, new wealth will flow through agricultural areas, even after a severe collapse. Operating as independent contractors in most rural areas won't be quite as easy as it was when I was young. Farm operations have grown tremendously in size and complexity these last few years. Dramatically fewer people live in rural areas, but this may change as retreaters return to the country.

However, dramatically more feed grains, heads of livestock, truck crops, and other products are produced out on our farms than even 10 years ago. Demand will remain high to insatiable, along with the fact that our rural economies are now technologically like giant watches. Huge numbers of very skilled people are required to keep that watch running correctly. Think of the fellow who keeps more than busy servicing milking machines. When I was young, we hired out milking cows by hand. Demand for dairy products has grown so large that we could not supply that demand by using hand-milking methods.

At any rate, let's conclude by noting that throughout life, especially during your later years, an ironclad rule of employment threes is essential, especially for rural survivor/retreaters.

CONCLUSION

Engaged, contemplative readers probably have one big question, as well as many lesser ones, regarding a valid, 21st-century survival plan. We already understand, within reasonable parameters, how to predict our coming economic collapse. And we know in broad, general terms what we must endure to survive that collapse. Exact, day-to-day retreating details are always a work in progress. Time and experience will eventually answer these smaller questions.

What has not been discussed is why we can probably count on a four- to six-year period before our society mends and what signs we can depend on as indicators that this mending is indeed taking place. These predictions are based on what we have seen, and are currently seeing, in many other countries around the world. Nothing much changes in this regard, although—as mentioned over and over—exact measures to deal with our new retreat realities have altered significantly from what we assumed them to be in the 1900s.

Before proceeding, it seems helpful to summarize what we already know, as well as the ironclad survival rules that we all must be aware of and implement.

1. Although it is seldom true when people say that things are different, it really is different this time because of the severity of the coming social and economic collapse, for which we must validly plan to hunker down for at least four to six years.
2. Survival rule of threes related to food, water, energy, med-

ical provisions, and shelter have not changed, but they have become much more difficult to implement successfully.
3. Because of the duration of a national collapse, coupled with a society that continues to believe a bankrupt government can supply their needs, city life will be brutal, accompanied by huge diebacks. It's no longer feasible to plan to hunker down for a year or two in the city until the crises pass.
4. We can be certain how all this will play out because of examples observed in at least 14 different countries around the world, many of which are way ahead of us in this economic collapse business.
5. Government rules and regulations, which almost certainly will be selectively enforced against rural retreaters, could possibly create great hardships for retreaters.
6. We can know with great precision when a collapse is imminent. This will occur when total government debt, both state and national, materially exceeds the total gross national product. When this line is crossed, government borrowing will exceed tax receipts, causing government to be unable to pay its bills. As is now true with Greek, Italian, and Spanish bonds, interest rates will then soar. When bond rates exceed 6 percent, collapse is imminent.
7. History instructs us that when total numbers of citizens who rely on government largesse exceed 50 percent, a country's economy shuts down.
8. Incidences of successful survival in cities will be unique and uncommon. Only those who move to rural areas and learn to live there have any real chance of making it.
9. Survivors/retreaters must make their move as soon as possible to accommodate what will be an extremely steep learning curve.
10. People who become refugees without a plan or place are dead meat.
11. Those who leave cities early can do so with most of their goods and plans intact.
12. Knowing what specific items might have value in a col-

lapsed economy is extremely difficult to predict. This is true even though we have numerous examples, including basket cases such as Cuba and the former Rhodesia.

13. An age-old philosophy suggests that skills and talents, especially in medical/dental areas, will be in great demand.
14. A retreat's best defense is deep obscurity and secrecy.
15. Armed defense of your retreat could engender severe social and legal problems that could compromise your situation. Don't do anything stupid, and remember the old adage: a battle avoided is a battle won.
16. Because of the long retreat duration envisioned, periodic resupply will be vitally important to retreaters.
17. Retreat mechanization will be necessary, or workloads will become insurmountable.
18. Out on rural retreats, if no chore is so pressing that it should have been done yesterday, you just don't understand the situation. The workload is formidable.
19. Cordial, longstanding relations with area farmers will be necessary in order to resupply.
20. Some movement in and out of a retreat will be necessary for resupply and other tasks. It is best to plan for transport vehicles and machinery necessary to move heavy goods economically.
21. Personal downsizing, including food and shelter, will be necessary. In many cases these will be much more severe than initially hoped or planned for.
22. Great economic accommodations must occur. Life will not continue on as in the past.
23. Recent changes in rural flora and fauna have made living off the land much more difficult. I know of no place left in this world where one can successfully live off the land. I have lived and worked in 95 different countries, mostly in rural settings, and I have never found even one place.
24. Traditional sources of income, such as government and personal pensions and Social Security benefits, will disappear or dramatically shrink.

25. Financial security requires that everyone have three distinct income-producing businesses or occupations, including ones for women and children over the age of 14 as part of their retreat economics.
26. Financial security during the declining years will also require three separate sources of income. It is much easier to establish these after people have spent their lives engaged in such a practice.
27. Citizens who live through our emerging crisis will be those who can produce a product or service of value.
28. Even in our 21st-century, impure, survival/retreat situations, survival rules of thermodynamics will apply. For example, we shouldn't expend more energy in undertaking a project—no matter how necessary—than is earned in that endeavor. Cutting firewood by hand, filing out tractor parts manually, and sport hunting are examples of activities that may expend too much energy for their contributions.
29. It is important to have nutritious, inexpensive, repetitious foods that you can tolerate at the retreat. If you stock only your favorite things, your supplies will dwindle too quickly, perhaps out of boredom. If you store food that you cannot eat because of allergies or intolerances, it does you no good.
30. Rural economies that currently produce huge quantities of food are technologically constructed like fine watches. Many skilled technicians are required to keep things running.
31. Rural economies are not closed. Great wealth comes from the soil. Employment in rural areas, especially as more and more folks move in, is both feasible and probable.
32. Employment, especially types that deploy vital skills, will integrate and ingratiate newcomers into rural economies.

This brings us to the final key question: why do we expect that our economy will return to some degree of normalcy and growth after four to six years? This is an especially good question, given that Japan's economy has remained mired in recession for more than 30 years, depending on how one counts and who is counting.

Conclusion

Then what will be some sure signs we, as a society, are mending? First, Japan's example is not a particularly good one. Japanese society is one of the most-regulated ones on Earth. For a short time, it produced some notable growth, which is not unusual among fascist economies. Freedom, as demonstrated over and over worldwide, leads to economic expansion. In the long run, a rising tide floats all ships. Japan's old society cannot and will not change.

North Korea and South Korea both started out at the same economic level in the late 1940s. South Korea is a long way from being a free country on a level with Hong Kong, Singapore, or Canada. Yet, today, average South Koreans earn and hold 20 times as much income and wealth as North Koreans.

President Ronald Reagan, with his freedom agenda, was able to steer us out of a Jimmy Carter–induced recession in only two years. Similarly, Great Britain under Margaret Thatcher corrected its economy in only three or four years. Germany under Gerhard Schröder took four or five years—depending on how you count—after it deregulated its labor markets. Sweden also underwent a quiet deregulation that helped it climb out of tough times. Currently the Swedes are justifiably proud of the fact that they are not part of the European economic collapse and that past economic/social reforms have been effective. Iceland is not out of the ice yet, but it has managed a dramatic turnaround in just over a year.

Looking at countries that devolved from communism is helpful. It took China (although still technically a communist state) six or eight years to move from starvation to prosperity, although this is still a work in progress. The Czech Republic, the Slovak Republic, Poland, the Baltic nations (Estonia, Latvia and Lithuania], East Germany, India, and Chile all moved rapidly—in six to eight years—into hugely more prosperous states than they were under communism or socialism.

In every one of these cases, the key was deregulation. This is now universally accepted. You want more farm production? Give farmers their fields and let them freely sell and produce for an open market. It happened in these countries so quickly that it was breathtaking. Currently Burma/Myanmar is just coming into enlightenment. It will be interesting to see how quickly that works out for that country and its people.

Estimating a four-to-six-year economic fix is just that—an estimate. Some knowledgeable people estimate it will take 10 years. Based on what we have seen worldwide, the time needed for an economic fix to work will be in direct proportion to the depths of the economic collapse. In other words, folks in general already know down in the depths of their souls that deregulation and freedom lead to prosperity. But some will try to game the system to the bitter end. A total, severe economic collapse wherein there is no place else to turn will force most of us to look again to traditional, workable engines of growth.

Pick your own number for the duration. Based on what we have experienced, four to six years certainly looks realistic. We will know we are on the mend economically when deregulation becomes a national passion, almost a sporting contest. I'd say real reform is under way when it is politically possible, and even popular, to set aside 10,000 rules and regulations per day for 30 days running; when entire government offices, bureaus, and cabinets are abolished; when thousands of bureaucrats are forced to find productive employment, thus allowing government spending to reduce to one-third of what it is now. Can't happen, you say? With no money to send, how is our cloud of locusts going to be able to buy food, shelter, and transportation?

Can we be optimistic about this happening in the United States? Definitely. Unlike Japan, Americans have freedom in our DNA.

Deregulation of a most basic, rudimentary nature is even being discussed in today's Italy, France, and Spain. This is not a misprint. Politicians in regulation-choked France are, according to a recent *Wall Street Journal* article, actually thinking about some deregulation of their labor markets. It is encouraging that people worldwide instinctively know that deregulation is the solution.

English politicians apparently are now recalling the successes of Margaret Thatcher. Britain's Labor government announced it will scrap thousands of regulations afflicting small- and medium-sized businesses. This is an attempt to allow new business start-ups to focus on creating more business, income, and jobs, according to John Vincent Cable, Britain's Secretary of State for Business, Innovation, and Skills.

In conclusion, based on experiences and movements in other counties, we can validly speculate that four to six years of trauma will do it for the United States. We also know that "the cure" is universally known and understood.

Some groups will try mightily to retain their privileged status as drones, living a good life off the public dole, but the depth of our collapse will quickly grind them out. Collapse is inevitable simply because there is no way to pay off the mountain of public debt we now face, and we cannot inflate our way out of this massive debt, as some policymakers suggest. Think of pre–World War II Germany, Mexico, Argentina, and Zimbabwe in this regard. Inflating our massive debt would certainly cause more problems than even Germany faced after World War I! Then as deregulation is achieved, our economy will again roll along nicely, creating new jobs, new technologies, new income, and new wealth for all willing to be producers.

That's our hope for 21st-century survival.

8874